MANAGING
Brain Injury

A Guide to Living Well
with Brain Injury

MANAGING
Brain Injury

A Guide to Living Well
with Brain Injury

Editors
Michael R. Yochelson, M.D.
Penny Wolfe, Ph.D.

Foreword by Bob Woodruff

NRH Press
Washington, D.C.

Copyright 2010
NRH Press

Paperback edition published by
NRH Press
National Rehabilitation Hospital
Publication Office
102 Irving Street, N.W.
Washington, D.C. 20010

Trade paperback ISBN 978-0-9661676-9-6

◊ ◊ ◊ ◊

Hardcover edition published by
ABI Professional Publications
P.O. Box 149
St. Petersburg, FL 33731

ISBN 978-1-886236-51-6

Dedication

*This book is dedicated to Bruce Ramsey, a survivor of a
severe traumatic brain injury, and his loving wife, Ellen Ramsey.
These two people have learned much about living with brain
injury over the years and have used this knowledge to
teach many others. They are dedicated to improving the lives of
people with brain injuries. They both sit on the Board of Directors
of the Brain Injury Association of DC. They work tirelessly to
advocate, educate, and provide the resources necessary for
people to be able to transition from injury back to an active,
productive, and meaningful life.*

*Thank you, Bruce and Ellen. You provide endless inspiration
to the Brain Injury Team at NRH!*

Acknowledgments

Each day every single team member at the National Rehabilitation Hospital (NRH) is "adding life to years." We hope that this book will provide information to survivors of brain injury and their families that will help to add life to their years.

We would like to thank all of the patients with whom we have worked over the years. It is you who provide the motivation to each of our staff to excel in the area of brain injury rehabilitation and to inspire the authors of this book to take the time and effort necessary to accomplish what they have.

We would like to thank NRH's President Emeritus, Mr. Edward A. Eckenhoff, without whose efforts and devotion, NRH would not exist to benefit the thousands of people who pass through its doors every year. The year that this book was written, 2009, was a major milestone for NRH as Mr. Eckenhoff has moved from President to President Emeritus, and Mr. John Rockwood has taken over as President and CEO of NRH. Also during this year, much thought has been given and actions taken to move toward increasing clinical and research opportunities in the area of brain injury. Publication of this book is very much a part of that effort. In addition to our gratitude toward our senior hospital executives, we would like to thank Dr. Edward Healton, the Senior Vice President for Medical Affairs, for his support.

We cannot thank enough each of the chapter authors of this book. Without them, we would not be publishing this book that will benefit thousands of persons with brain injury and their loved ones.

We also wish to thank Mr. Robert Hartmann for providing the administrative support necessary and the commitment to keep us driving forward with writing, editing, and publishing the book. We would like to thank Emily Turk for advice on editing and interviewing many patients to provide quotes throughout the book. Also, she wrote an entire section dedicated to the real-life stories of our patients. Also, we thank Mr. Art Brown, our publisher, without whose guidance this book would not be such a success.

Finally, we would like to thank our families and friends without whose support and forgiveness for the late nights and weekends away, this book would not have happened. Michael would especially like to thank Guy Parker for his unwavering encouragement and his mother, Judy Yochelson, for her editorial assistance. Penny would like to thank her mother, Linda Wolfe, for editorial assistance and her friends and family for their patience and understanding.

Contributors

Heather Campbell, C.T.R.S.
Recreation Therapist
National Rehabilitation Hospital
Washington, D.C.

**Alison Cuneo, P.T., D.P.T.,
N.C.S.**
Resource Physical Therapist
National Rehabilitation Hospital
Washington, D.C.

Inbal Eshel, M.A., C.C.C.-SLP
Speech-Language Pathologist
Performance Measure Analyst
MedStar Research Institute
University of Maryland
College Park, Maryland

**William Garmoe, Ph.D.,
A.B.P.P.-C.N.**
Coordinator, Neuropsychology
   Services
Investigator, Neurosciences
   Research Center
National Rehabilitation Hospital
Washington, D.C.

Olivia Glover, B.S., O.T.R/L
Senior Occupational Therapist
National Rehabilitation Hospital
Washington, D.C.

**Jennifer Davies Hendricks,
M.S.W., L.I.C.S.W.**
AVP, Referrals and Case
   Management
National Rehabilitation Hospital
Washington, D.C.

**Susan T. Kaufmann, M.A.,
Ed.S.**
Educational Program Specialist
U.S. Department of Education
Office of Special Education
   Programs
Washington, D.C.

**Kimberly Lockett, M.S.W.,
L.I.C.S.W., C.B.I.S.**
Case Manager
National Rehabilitation Hospital
Washington, D.C.

**Rhoda Onyima, M.S.N.,
C.R.N.P.**
Nurse Practitioner
National Rehabilitation Hospital
Washington, D.C.

Kelly Peterson, O.T.D.
Occupational Therapist
WakeMed Rehab
Raleigh, North Carolina

Cynthia G. Pineda, M.D., F.A.A.P.M.& R.
Associate Program Director
GUH-NRH PMR
Residency Training Program
National Rehabilitation Hospital
Washington, D.C.

Judson Richardson, M.S.W., L.I.C.S.W.
Social Worker
National Rehabilitation Hospital
Washington, D.C.

Neepa Shah, M.S., O.T.R/L
Clinical Supervisor, Occupational
Therapy
National Rehabilitation Hospital
Washington, D.C.

Brownrigg Snow, M.S.
Senior Speech Language
Pathologist
National Rehabilitation Hospital
Washington, D.C.

Tresa Roebuck Spencer, Ph.D., A.B.P.P.-C.N.
Neuropsychologist
University of Oklahoma
Oklahoma City, Oklahoma

Penny L. Wolfe, Ph.D.
Clinical Neuropsychologist
Co-Director, Brain Injury Program
National Rehabilitation Hospital
Washington, D.C.

Michael R. Yochelson, M.D.
Associate Medical Director
Neurological Programs
National Rehabilitation Hospital
Washington, D.C.

Lauren M. Zimmerman-Thomas, Psy.D.
Neuropsychology Postdoctoral
Resident
National Rehabilitation Hospital
Washington, D.C.

Contents

Foreword

Bob Woodruff

Before I was injured, I had never thought much about head injuries at all. I didn't know anyone who had suffered a head injury or brain injury, didn't think a great deal about wearing a helmet while skiing or biking, and never contemplated the possibilities of being permanently impaired.

In my line of work as a journalist who covered wars and areas of conflict, there were two outcomes I could foresee—making it back home or being killed in the field.

On January 29, 2006, the unexpected happened, and my life and my family's life changed dramatically. I was heading down a road in Taji, Iraq, on the top of an Iraqi APC (armored personnel carrier). This was my seventh trip to this country, but the first time we were reporting about the collaboration between United States and Iraqi forces against the insurgents.

In an instant, an improvised explosive device (IED) exploded about 20 yards from the vehicle, injuring me as well as my cameraman, Doug Vogt. The force of the blast, a 155-mm shell, resulted in a bleed on the left temporal lobe. Hundreds of rocks, packed around the IED, were blasted into the side of my face, chin, and neck.

As they do every day in these wars, Army medics flew us by helicopter to Baghdad and then on to Balad, where within the hour, 16 cm of my skull were removed as my brain continued to swell. For the next 36 days, I remained in a medically induced coma, but the quick actions and amazing skill of the medics, military doctors, nurses, and assistants not only saved my life, but also my brain function following this life-threatening injury.

From Balad I was sent to the military's Regional Medical Center in Landstuhl, Germany, a major way station for wounded soldiers en route to the United States. Just 60 hours after my family arrived to see me there, I was ready to be transported again to neurosurgical care at Bethesda Naval Hospital outside Washington, D.C. It was there that I received top-notch medical care from an expert team of dedicated military specialists. It was their skill, perseverance, team approach, and kindness that created a platform from which to heal.

Once I passed through the acute stage of my injury, the real work began in my long journey toward healing during rehabilitation. Time, energy, commitment, and dedicated professionals supplied the framework to help my brain heal. The therapists, doctors, and nurses in rehab were some of the finest, most patient and motivating people I have ever met. I will always be indebted to them. The love and encouragement of family and friends were invaluable, and it challenged and spurred me every day to "get my brain back."

A brain injury is a life-altering experience. For some, the changes are subtle, hidden. For others, the differences can be more dramatic, causing alterations in personality, thought, and movement that are permanent. For every one of the brain injured, there is hopefully a dedicated and loving caregiver — spouse, parent, sibling, child, or friend — who is advocating, praying, hoping, and believing that we will have a good outcome, despite the grim prognosis.

In the United States and in the wars in Iraq and Afghanistan, we are faced with a wave of wounded, many of them young, all of them returning to a life vastly different from what they left. Families must learn to deal with a new reality surrounding brain injuries. No one predicted there would be so many injured in this war. The current statistics are that more than 360,000 individuals have some form of a brain injury, which can range from the most severe traumatic brain injuries (TBI) to closed head injury and post-traumatic stress disorder (PTSD). Like me, many of these warriors had never heard about TBI. Very few knew that here at home roughly 1.5 million Americans receive a brain injury each year and 5.4 million are living with brain injuries. The increase of injuries from the war is bringing the issue to the forefront. Military and civilian doctors are working and collaborating together like never before.

We will never be able to eradicate brain injuries from humanity. We will always have accidents, injuries, violence, and the unpredictability of life. But one thing that can ease the journey is a book like *Managing Brain Injury: A Guide to Living Well with Brain Injury*. This book offers patients and families practical, useful information and helps to make some sense out of what is often, especially initially, a senseless situation.

The brain injury experts at National Rehabilitation Hospital (NRH) have drawn on their years of clinical experience to help patients and caregivers cope with the process of rehabilitation. It's a realistic look at what patients and families can expect throughout the journey, and it is filled with critical tools to help ease the anxiety they will no doubt face following brain injury. Especially helpful are the personal stories of hope from men and women who have suffered brain injury, moved through the rehabilitative process, and successfully rebuilt their lives. I applaud NRH for compiling such a critical resource.

I am incredibly blessed to have had such a remarkable recovery. I am well aware that my outcome is not the norm. Although I still suffer from mild aphasia (the inability to retrieve certain words), in particular when I am tired, I have been able to return to work at ABC News as a reporter and anchor. I lead a full life with very few daily reminders of the trauma we all endured as a family. I am a walking miracle, as so many have called me, and I am a testament to the power of the brain, the value of intensive rehabilitation, the love of family, and the resiliency of the human spirit.

Bob Woodruff

Introduction

More than 5 million Americans live with disability caused by a traumatic brain injury (TBI). That number grows if you include other (nontraumatic) causes of brain injury. At National Rehabilitation Hospital (NRH) in Washington, D.C., we strive to provide the best rehabilitative care available for these people so that they can return to a life as independent as possible. This book was written by the staff at NRH to serve as a resource for survivors of brain injury and their families and caregivers.

The decade from 1990 through 1999 was declared "The Decade of the Brain" by the U.S. Congress. These words clearly indicate the importance of the brain as well as the urgency for the research and medical establishments to develop and provide cutting-edge treatments for people who have brain disease or injury. The brain is the control center for the body, so injury to the brain can have a negative impact on almost every system in the body. Additionally, brain injury has a direct influence on a person's ability to function in society because of changes in language, cognition (thinking), emotion, and behavior.

TBI affects more than just the survivor of the injury. It affects his or her loved ones, friends, and entire social network. This observation has recently been brought to the forefront of American politics because of the number of brain injuries incurred by service members serving our country in Operation Iraqi Freedom and Operation Enduring Freedom (in Afghanistan).

This book focuses on the moderate to severely injured person who may have very significant impairment. It reviews the acute rehabilitation process in detail. It also provides information that will be useful for persons with brain injuries and their caregivers to keep as a reference for months and years after the injury. Although not all of the information will apply directly to people with mild TBI, even those people living with a mild brain injury will find useful information in the book. The same applies to nontraumatic brain injury. While not all of the information applies to people who have suffered a nontraumatic injury, much of it will.

It should be noted that the term, "person who has suffered a brain injury," or similar term is used throughout this text, rather than "patient" in most cases. This conscious decision was made by our team of authors because these people will be living with the brain injury for the rest of their lives, but will not necessarily be a patient (in the hospital) when they are reading this book.

It is the philosophy of NRH that through rehabilitation we are "adding life to years." Whether you are a brain injury survivor, family member, employer, friend, or someone else who has contact with people with brain injuries, we hope that you find the information in this book very useful to you. As medical care and emergency services in the United States improves, it is likely that we will see more people who survive brain injuries and we will need to learn how to help them. We also need to do more to advocate for survivors so that they receive the services they need. One of the most important aspects of brain injury rehabilitation is patient and caregiver education. This book is one small part of that process. We are pleased to be able to share our knowledge and experiences with you to help anyone who has suffered from a brain injury to achieve an improved quality of life.

Michael R. Yochelson, M.D., Editor
Medical Director
Brain Injury Programs
National Rehabilitation Hospital
Washington, D.C.

Penny Wolfe, Ph.D., Editor
Co-Director
Brain Injury Programs
National Rehabilitation Hospital
Washington, D.C.

A Leaf of Knowledge

I don't know
what the doctor means by "mostly"
within the radiation field
I don't know
for how long I will need this cane
I don't know
what the scan will look like one month,
four months,
four years from now.

All I know is the air I breathe in this instant—
spring's sweet whisper—
into my lungs,
my friend at my side,
his broad hand between my shoulder-blades,
the living God,
the love of my friends and family,
and the warm skin of her knee
onto which I lay my cheek, to sleep.

—Brendan Ogg

1

THE BRAIN

MICHAEL R. YOCHELSON

*After his injury, we were Christopher's [my son's] brain,
his voice, his hands and legs.* —Maryann Griswold

The brain is the control center of the body. It allows you to see, taste, hear, think, and touch. It also controls voluntary and involuntary movements. Furthermore, it controls many necessary functions for life that you do not even have to think about, such as breathing, heart rate, bladder control, etc. The brain is also responsible for emotions and behaviors, such as happiness, sadness, aggression, and anxiety.

THE NORMAL BRAIN

The brain itself is very soft. It is protected both by a hard skull as well as a fluid, cerebrospinal fluid (CSF), which acts as a shock absorber. In very basic terms you can divide the brain into the brainstem, cerebellum, and cerebral hemispheres (cerebrum). The hemispheres are further divided into the outer portion, or cortex, and the deeper structures (e.g., thalamus, hippocampus, basal ganglia, etc.), some of which will be discussed later.

The brainstem is the lower, narrow portion of your brain located just above the spinal cord. This part of your brain controls many basic functions required to live. These functions are referred to as autonomic function and include breathing, blood pressure, and heart rate. Some of the basic functions of the head and neck, such as eye movement and swallowing, are controlled in part by the brainstem. Sleep and arousal are also controlled by structures in the brainstem.

The cortex is made up of four areas called the frontal, parietal, temporal, and occipital lobes. All four lobes are present on both sides of the

1

brain. The term "hemisphere" refers to the entire cortex (all four lobes) on one side of the brain. For the most part, the brain controls the opposite side of the body. So, for example, the left frontal cortex is involved in the movements of the right side of the body. However, there are differences between the two hemispheres as will be discussed later.

There are many other specific functions of the cortex. These functions are too complex to discuss in detail in this book. The following is just a single example of function from each cortical lobe to demonstrate the variability of function. The occipital lobe is involved with vision; the parietal lobe with visuo-spatial orientation; the temporal lobe with memory; and the frontal lobe with behavior. However, it is also important to note that many functions are controlled by multiple areas of the brain, so while the temporal lobe is important for the control of memory, problems with memory result from damage to other areas of the brain as well.

Some of the more specific functions of the brain are discussed below and organized by location.

Frontal Lobe

The frontal lobe controls gross motor control, such as moving the arms or walking. (See Figure 1.1.) It takes information from several areas of the brain to perform complex tasks; this is called executive function. Executive function requires the ability to plan and organize. Here is an example of executive function: Jennifer senses hunger and is able to recognize the need to eat; she then takes the initiative to go to the kitchen, make a sandwich, and eat it.

The frontal lobe contains Broca's area that is necessary for normal speech and language function. Specifically, it controls the motor control of speaking. An impairment in Broca's area causes one to have difficulty speaking even though the person may know what he or she wants to say and can understand other people when they speak.

Initiation is the person's ability to start a process. This may be a simple movement or a complex task, such as getting dressed; it may be the process of starting to speak or promptly responding to a question. The frontal lobe functions to initiate actions without an external prompt. There may be problems with both initiation and executive function. If this is the situation, the person with the brain injury may need verbal or visual cues, not only to start the task, but instructions on individual steps. An example would be a person initiating getting dressed in the morning. If the person has poor initiation, someone may need to say, "get dressed." If the person has poor initiation and executive function, someone may have to go through the process step by step to get the brain-injured person dressed.

This part of the brain is also responsible for inhibiting inappropriate behavior. This area helps people to control their behavior in a manner that is socially appropriate. When the frontal lobe is injured and the person cannot maintain appropriate behavior (e.g., cursing, inappropriate sexual behavior, etc.), this is referred to as "disinhibition."

The frontal lobe is involved with the outward expression of emotion (affect). Often after a TBI, especially if the frontal lobe was involved, the person may have a very "flat affect" in which he or she shows only limited expression of emotion and appears depressed, even if he is not.

Parietal Lobe

Much of the job of the parietal lobe is integrating sensory input from other parts of the brain. (See Figure 1.1.) While the thalamus is the primary integrator of sensory signals, the parietal lobe receives these signals and processes them so the person responds accordingly. It turns a basic signal, like touch, pain, or temperature, into a more meaningful signal such as recognizing that his or her left leg is hanging off the side of the bed or that there is a dime in his or her right hand. It is also a key component in visuo-spatial perception. This is quite important in routine function. It allows one to fully attend to their surroundings.

Temporal Lobe

The temporal lobe contains centers for hearing, taste, and smell; it is important for the integration of the sensory signals to other areas of the brain. (See Figure 1.1.) It plays a key role in memory and language function. Wernicke's area is at the temporo-parietal junction. This area controls comprehension of language. This lobe is also involved in control of emotions.

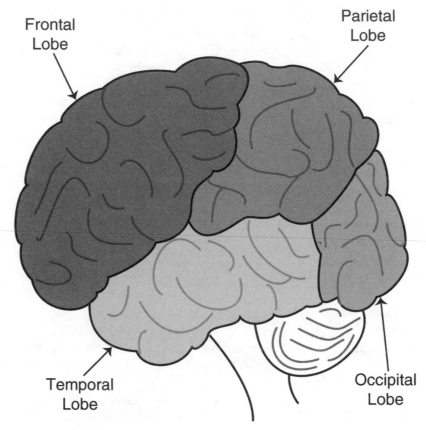

Figure 1.1 The four lobes of the brain's cortex.

Occipital Lobe

The occipital lobe is the location of both the primary visual cortex as well as association cortex which is integral in the processing of images. (See Figure 1.1.) However, to get to the occipital lobe at the back of the brain, the visual pathway runs through all of the other lobes. Therefore, vision problems could occur from injury to many different areas of the brain.

Cerebellum

The cerebellum sends signals to the cortex and other areas of the brain and receives information from the spinal cord and some of the deeper

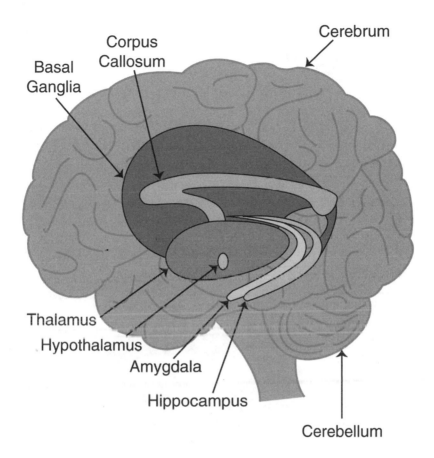

Figure 1.2 The basal ganglia, cerebellum, and deep structures of the brain.

brain structures permitting coordination of movement, balance, and the ability to remain upright. (See Figure 1.2.) The middle of the cerebellum is key for balance and walking. The cerebellar hemispheres do more to control the smooth movement of the arms and legs. The cerebellum, however, is critical for things other than just balance and coordination. The cerebellum also plays an important role in cognition.

Thalamus

All sensory input goes through the thalamus. (See Figure 1.2.) This is the primary relay area for all sensory signals. The thalamus receives the sensory input from the nerves in the arms and legs that travel up the spinal cord through the brainstem to the thalamus. From there, they are directed to the appropriate part of the brain, primarily the cortex. The thalamus also receives other sensory signals, such as smell.

In addition to its primary responsibility of processing sensory signals, the thalamus is involved in integrating these signals for abstract thinking and goal-directed behaviors. The thalamus also plays a roll in attention, memory, and learning because of its connections with the hippocampus.

Basal Ganglia

The basal ganglia are located deep in the brain. (See Figure 1.2.) They, like the thalamus, are considered "subcortical" structures. They help control movement. Although the frontal lobe controls gross movement, one cannot perform smooth, accurate movements without the basal ganglia functioning normally.

Brainstem

The brainstem has many key roles in sustaining life as mentioned above. It also contains the control center (nuclei) for all of the cranial nerves. The cranial nerves control many activities involving the head and neck, for example vision, hearing, taste, swallowing, and facial movement and sensation.

KEY POINTS

- The brain is divided into four lobes plus the cerebellum, brainstem, and deep structures, such as the thalamus.
- Each area of the brain has its own function resulting in different symptoms if injured.

2

TRAUMATIC BRAIN INJURY

MICHAEL R. YOCHELSON

. . . I'm running as fast as I can towards the finish line, tied at the ankle to someone who keeps falling asleep! Sometimes we are both running, but most of the time I am just dragging her along.
—Anonymous

Traumatic brain injury (TBI) is a major cause of disability in the United States. Each year over 1.4 million Americans suffer a brain injury. The majority of these injuries are mild; however, approximately 10% are moderate and 10% are severe. Because many people who have survived a brain injury are left with permanent impairment, it is estimated that there are more than 5 million Americans who are disabled as a result of a TBI. Among the people who have had a mild TBI, about 85% will have no long-term problems. The remaining people may have persistent symptoms. The most common symptoms are headaches, dizziness, and cognitive difficulties, such as memory impairment. Other symptoms that may result from a mild injury include fatigue, difficulties with sleep, and emotional or behavioral problems. Physical impairment is uncommon in this population. These persistent symptoms after a mild TBI may be referred to as postconcussive syndrome.

The most common causes of TBI are falls and motor vehicle accidents. Alcohol is the number one indirect cause. In other words, when people are using alcohol, they have a much greater risk of suffering a brain injury because they fall or get in an accident. Also, someone else who is drinking alcohol and driving could hit an innocent person, resulting in a TBI.

Most people who have had a mild TBI do not require hospitalization. Most severe injuries require medical attention and often prolonged hospitalization, to include surgery, intensive care services, and inpatient rehabilitation.

INJURIES TO THE BRAIN

The brain can be injured a number of different ways, some of which will be discussed below. However, in addition to these, acquired (nontraumatic) brain injury can come from infections and other disease processes.

Skull Fractures

Skull fractures occur when a blow to the head is hard enough to break the skull. Sometimes a skull fracture can happen without any piece of the skull moving and pressing against the brain. In such cases, the fracture heals by itself. When the skull moves and presses against the brain, it causes further injury, bleeding, and the need for treatment. In the case where there is no movement of the skull, there can be a "head injury" without a "brain injury." Whenever there is involvement of the brain itself, the term "brain injury" should be used to distinguish these entities.

Contusions

Contusions are a bruising of the brain. Contusions often occur when the brain shifts under the skull, hitting against the inner walls of the skull, thus causing a bruise. The damage of a contusion can be serious, requiring treatment. Often after a traumatic brain injury, there will be multiple contusions. Common types of contusion are "coup" and "contrecoup" injuries. The coup injury occurs in the brain where the skull contacted a hard object. The contrecoup injury occurs on the opposite side of the brain (see Figure 2.1).

Concussion

Concussions involve a brief loss or alteration of consciousness after a blow to the brain. There may be a short time of memory loss and ongo-

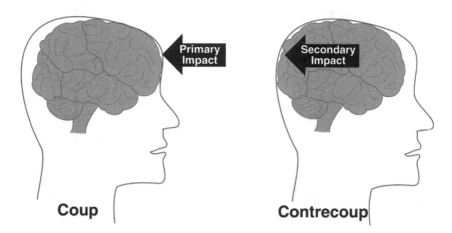

Figure 2.1 Coup and contrecoup injuries to the brain.

ing headache. In more serious cases, concussions can lead to weakness, longer memory loss, and paralysis.

Blast Injuries

A type of brain injury that is being seen more commonly as a result of modern warfare is the blast injury. A brain injury caused by a blast is often seen following detonation of an IED (improvised explosive device) or RPG (rocket-propelled grenade). Additionally, we are seeing blast injuries following explosives and building collapse used in terrorist acts, such as the terrorist attack and collapse of the World Trade Center. These injuries can occur from direct trauma to the brain (similar to a contusion) or from a person hitting his head during the blast. However, there is additional damage from the blast wave itself as it is transmitted through the brain.

Hematomas

Hematomas occur when a blow to the head ruptures one or more of the blood vessels, leading to bleeding or leaking of blood from the vessel. Sometimes hematomas result from a skull fracture or a sharp object penetrating the brain and causing bleeding. There are various kinds of hematomas: epidural hematomas, subdural hematomas, intracranial hematomas. These hematomas may also occur without trauma, for example, a ruptured aneurysm.

Diffuse Axonal Injury

Diffuse axonal injury (DAI) is damage to the white matter deep in the brain as a result of shearing forces from rotation or rapid deceleration of the head just after impact. There are usually multiple areas of DAI in the brain. DAI can be seen on MRI, but is rarely appreciated on a CT scan. However, even with MRI using standard techniques, DAI can be missed. Newer techniques, such as diffusion tensor imaging, which can see injury at a microscopic level, are better at picking up diffuse axonal injury. Because DAI is injury to the myelin that covers the axons in the brain, it causes a loss of ability of the nerve axons to communicate with one another; in other words, it decreases the effectiveness of signals being transmitted throughout the brain. It can affect many different functions in the brain.

Anoxia

Anoxia happens when there is a lack of oxygen to the brain. While this is generally a nontraumatic type of brain injury, occasionally as a result of trauma, a person can go into shock and, therefore, also have an anoxic brain injury. When the brain does not get enough oxygen, brain cells become damaged or die. Anoxia often occurs as a result of a heart attack. When the heart stops beating, there is decreased or absent blood flow to the brain and, therefore, the oxygen supply to the brain is significantly diminished.

SEIZURES

Following a brain injury, one is at increased risk for seizures. The actual risk is not that high, but it is still important to be aware of this fact. A seizure is an abnormal electrical discharge that occurs in the injured part of the brain. Epilepsy is recurrent seizures. It can cause many different types of symptoms. A common symptom is twitching, jerking or other uncontrollable movements. These movements may occur in just one arm or one leg, on one side of the body, or on both sides. It can even just be twitching in the face. Seizures may also result in loss of consciousness or a change in the level of consciousness. A person who is seizing may stare into space and one cannot get his or her attention. There are many other symptoms of seizures, but these are the most common. A "grand mal" seizure is one in which a person loses consciousness and has shaking in both arms and legs. Sometimes the person seizing may have incontinence (urinate on himself or herself) and/or bite his or her tongue. Most seizures will last from about 15 seconds to 2 minutes. If a seizure continues beyond several minutes, it may not stop on its own and someone should call 911 to get the person to an emergency room. He or she may need medications to stop the seizure. However, for anyone with known seizures who has a seizure typical for him or her, going to the emergency department is not usually necessary. Always discuss this with the doctor treating the seizures.

During a seizure, DO NOT PANIC. It is important to actually watch a clock to see how long it lasts because it may seem like eternity even if it only lasts a minute. Get the person to a safe place (e.g., lying on a bed or floor), make sure the head is protected during convulsions, turn the patient on his or her side if there is vomiting and DO NOT put anything in the mouth.

Most people only need to be on seizure medications for the first week after a traumatic brain injury. Certain groups of patients, for example, those with a gunshot wound with bullet fragments, may need to be on medications for a longer period of time since their risk for seizures is higher. Anti-seizure medications are also often prescribed for longer periods after non-traumatic brain injuries, particularly for people with brain tumors. There are many medications that are used to treat seizures. (See Chapter 9.) It is very important that the patient does not miss any doses of his or her medicine. Never stop a seizure medication without talking to the doctor first.

Some things lower the seizure threshold. This means that they increase the likelihood of having a seizure. These include alcohol and sleep deprivation. There are certain medications that lower the seizure threshold. There are also some medications that interact with the seizure medicine and may increase or decrease the level, putting the patient at risk of seizures. Therefore, it is important to let all physicians who treat the person with a brain injury know about the seizure risk and the list of medications that he or she is taking.

For anyone who has had a seizure, he or she will likely need to be on life-long medicine to prevent future seizures. Every state in the United States has laws about driving with seizures. Check with the local Motor Vehicle Administration to find out the specific laws in your state. Additional precautions should be taken to protect people who have seizures. These include no swimming alone, no working on ladders or at heights, and, in general avoiding any activity in which a sudden loss of consciousness or seizure would cause harm to the person with the seizure or others around him or her.

RANCHO LOS AMIGOS SCALE

The Rancho Los Amigos Cognitive Functioning Scale ("Rancho") is named for the Rancho Los Amigos National Rehabilitation Hospital in Los Angeles where it was developed in 1970 and is still frequently used today. The scale has been more recently revised to have 10 levels of cognitive functioning. (See below.) This scale is often used to determine whether a person who has had a brain injury is appropriate for a specific level of rehabilitation. However, it is not typically discussed on a regular basis within the rehabilitation team or with the patient and caregivers because the Rancho level does not indicate specific functional impairment. So, in the rehabilitation setting, it is much more useful for the team to evaluate the person's specific functions, using measures such as the Functional Independence Measure (FIM) or other tools. Nonetheless, the Rancho is one scale that is useful to understand as it demonstrates the different stages of recovery from a brain injury. It should be noted, however, that not every person goes through each level. Some people will start at a higher level; some may skip levels and others may fluctuate back and forth between levels. It is not unusual for someone to be at level 5 one day and level 4 the next; this situation does not imply that there is a problem. The scale is as follows:

- *Level 1: No response.* Patient appears to be in a very deep sleep or coma and does not respond to noise, touch, light, or sound.
- *Level 2: Generalized response.* Patient may move around, but the movement does not have any purpose. The person may open his

or her eyes, but does not seem to focus on anything.

- *Level 3: Localized response.* Patient may move his or her head to look at people or things. He or she may be able to follow one step, simple commands inconsistently.
- *Level 4: Confused and agitated.* Patient is very confused and becomes easily upset when there is too much noise or too much activity. He or she may be restless, aggressive, or verbally abusive. When the patient talks, it may not make sense.
- *Level 5: Confused and inappropriate.* Patient is still confused and conversations may still may not make sense. There can still be agitation during this phase, especially during stressful situations. There may be some return of memory, but large gaps remain; these gaps may become frustrating to the patient.
- *Level 6: Confused but appropriate.* Patient is still confused and needs directions on what to do or not to do. Many daily automatic tasks such as bathing, dressing, and brushing teeth start to become easier. Learning new tasks may still be difficult.
- *Level 7: Automatic and appropriate.* Patient can perform daily care needs and usually makes sense. There may still be small cognitive problems, but daily tasks can be managed. The ability to solve problems and make good decisions is developing and generally satisfactory in basic, familiar situations, but may be more difficult when adjusting to novel, complex situations.
- *Level 8: Purposeful and appropriate.* Patient is alert and oriented and can recall and integrate past events, learn new activities, and function in many activities without supervision. Patient is independent in home and living skills, may be capable of driving, yet still has poor stress tolerance, difficulties with judgment and abstract reasoning. Patient may function at a reduced level in society.
- *Level 9: Purposeful and appropriate with standby assist upon request.* Patient is aware of impairments and able to compensate. Patient is able to self-monitor behavior and may begin to be integrated into the community.
- *Level 10: Purposeful and appropriate at a modified independent level.* Patient demonstrates consistent behavior in social situations. His or her ability to think about consequences is intact, but may be slow. Workplace integration may be possible in this stage.

KEY POINTS

- Over 1.4 million Americans suffer a traumatic brain injury each year. The majority are mild, but approximately 10% are severe and 50,000 each year result in death.
- The most common causes of traumatic brain injury are falls and motor vehicle accidents; alcohol is the most common indirect cause.

3

NONTRAUMATIC BRAIN INJURY

MICHAEL R. YOCHELSON

*A catastrophic brain injury, multiple surgeries, extended hospital
stays, aggressive therapies to achieve a set of goals, a faith journey,
and having to relearn everything to become independent again, has
been a transformation of trials into triumphs.* —Selina Brijsbaji

When people think about brain
injury, usually their first thought is traumatic brain injury, or TBI. While
TBI is the focus of this book, it is important to discuss nontraumatic
brain injury as well. There are a number of ways to get a brain injury
that do not result from trauma. As a group, these injuries may be
referred to as acquired brain injury, or ABI. These are distinct from
developmental brain disorders that occur at or before birth and degen-
erative brain disorders that occur later in life, such as Alzheimer's disease, multiple sclerosis, and various other neurological diseases that
affect the brain. The hallmark of an acquired brain injury is that the
onset is sudden and usually occurs at a single point in time, rather than
a progressive process. However, some conditions, such as brain tumors,
are considered a type of acquired brain injury even though they may be
progressive. However, brain tumors cause an external insult to the brain
rather than a brain disease, which is why they present clinically more
like an acquired brain injury. Because of the potentially progressive
nature of brain tumors and their clinical variability based on the type of
tumor, these tumors will be discussed separately in the next chapter.
Other acquired brain injuries include bleeds from aneurysms or other
vascular problems, encephalitis, anoxic brain injury, and stroke. Some
people who have suffered a stroke present more as a typical "brain
injury," which is why we will discuss it briefly in this section. However,

for people who have suffered a stroke, another reference that may be helpful is *Managing Stroke: A Guide to Living Well After Stroke.* (See the References section for complete reference information.)

HEMORRHAGES

Bleeds into the brain, often termed CNS (central nervous system) bleeds, can occur for several reasons. An aneurysm is a ballooning of a blood vessel that causes thinning of the vessel wall and risk for rupture and bleeding. Most aneurysms have been present for years, and possibly since birth, prior to rupturing. Often there is no warning sign before the bleed. Some people, however, will have small bleeds before the major bleed. These small bleeds (called sentinel bleeds) may present as occasional, severe headaches. Once the aneurysm ruptures, the person experiencing this may have a severe headache, frequently described as "the worst headache of my life." The bleed may also be associated with seizures, altered mental status, loss of consciousness, and/or focal neurological symptoms, such as weakness. Depending on the size of the bleed, someone with an aneurysm rupture may have to undergo surgery to evacuate the blood to avoid increased pressure on the brain and help prevent further damage to the brain. Most people with an aneurysm rupture will also need some interventional procedures (i.e., through a catheter under radiographic guidance, not opening the skull) to remove the aneurysm or try to reduce the risk of having it rebleed. In addition to the congenital aneurysms that were mentioned above, people can develop "post-traumatic aneurysms" following a traumatic brain injury. This situation puts someone with a TBI at increased risk for bleeding. These are uncommon, but can occur.

In addition to aneurysms, there are other types of vascular problems that can lead to CNS bleeds. These include AVMs (arteriovenous malformations). These are almost always congenital. These are "tangles" of blood vessels that occur when the artery connects directly to veins without the capillaries in between. This condition puts patients at risk of bleeding because of the pressure change between the artery and vein. Due to the size or location of an AVM, they can cause neurological problems, such as seizures, fainting, or headaches even if they do not rupture. They are also at risk for rupture, like an aneurysm. Smaller AVMs have a higher risk for bleeding than do the larger ones; this is thought to be because they have a higher pressure in the arteries that send blood to the AVM. Once they rupture, the bleed can cause significant neurological impairment.

Aneurysms and AVMs are the two most common vascular lesions that will bleed. Also, other types of vascular malformations may bleed, including cavernous angiomas and venous angiomas. The different types of vascular malformations have different risks of bleeding, but once they do bleed, may have very similar clinical presentations.

In addition to aneurysms and other vascular malformations, hemorrhages may result from other problems, such as vasculitis. This problem can be caused by infectious or autoimmune causes or can be a primary CNS vasculitis. Hemorrhages may occur in the area of brain that has recently suffered a stroke. In the elderly, amyloid angiopathy is a common cause of hemorrhages. Deposits of a protein called amyloid in the walls of blood vessels make the elderly susceptible to bleeding and will often cause recurrent bleeds. Certain types of brain tumors also have a high incidence of bleeding. This type of tumor can cause brain injury, not only from the tumor itself, but from the bleeding as well as swelling and mass effect.

ANOXIC BRAIN INJURY

The brain needs oxygen to function and survive. Any loss of oxygen to the brain results in a brain injury. This injury can be referred to as a hypoxic brain injury if there is decreased, but not complete, loss of oxygen or anoxic brain injury if there is complete loss. Usually the loss of oxygen is caused by decreased blood flow to the brain, such as can occur if someone is having a cardiac arrest or in a drowning. It can also occur if the blood itself is not carrying sufficient oxygen as can be seen with a pulmonary embolism (blood clot to the lung) or pulmonary insufficiency from other causes.

Anoxic brain injuries are probably more like traumatic brain injuries than any of the acquired brain injuries discussed in this chapter. This is, in large part, because it affects multiple areas of the brain, rather than a focal area as is the case in stroke or brain tumors. The prognosis after anoxic brain injury is variable depending on the how long the brain did not get sufficient oxygen. Although variable, as a rule the prognosis after an anoxic brain injury is not as good as after a traumatic brain injury.

Nonetheless, people who have suffered an anoxic brain injury can still benefit from rehabilitation. It is best to discuss the prognosis with the doctors who can provide more specific information about this situation depending upon the medical history of a given person.

Movement disorders, such as tremors, myoclonus, and ataxia, are more prevalent among people with anoxic brain injuries. Sometimes these disorders respond to some medications or to therapy, but severe movement disorders can be very difficult to control and therapy may need to concentrate on ways to compensate for the problem.

Memory is another problem for these people. The hippocampus, part of the brain responsible for short-term memory, is highly susceptible to damage resulting in hypoxia or anoxia. Memory may improve with time, but there are no treatments that specifically treat this problem. As with the movements, the best rehabilitation involves helping the person to learn to manage through use of compensatory means.

ENCEPHALOPATHY

Encephalopathy is the disturbance of brain function that typically affects mental status and is frequently associated with seizures. There are many causes of encephalopathy. Sometimes the terms, encephalopathy and encephalitis, are used interchangeably. Encephalopathy is a broader term that describes brain function. An encephalitis may cause an encephalopathy, but it specifically refers to an inflammatory process in the brain that is commonly caused by an infection. The most common causes are viral encephalitides (viral encephalitis). Most of the time, a viral encephalitis does not require treatment and will resolve spontaneously. However, one of the most common ones that must be treated is herpes encephalitis (HSV encephalitis), which can be fatal if not treated, but responds well to treatment. However, even when treated with antiviral medications, the patient may still require some rehabilitation. Many other viruses cause encephalitis, but we do not have medicines to treat them. Bacterial encephalitis can also be fatal and, therefore, must be diagnosed and treated promptly. As with the viral encephalitis, after a bacterial encephalitis one may require rehabilitation. The course of recovery can be very prolonged. Other types of encephalitis may be autoimmune, that is, that the body produces an antibody in response to something external and this antibody ends up causing an encephalitis.

In addition to the encephalitis, an encephalopathy may be a result of a metabolic problem. Usually this occurs in the midst of other illnesses, such as liver or kidney disease. Treating the underlying problem is always the first step in treating an encephalopathy. Beyond that, management includes treating seizures, if present, and other medications to help with arousal, confusion, hallucinations, agitation, or other problems that may occur.

STROKE

Stroke is by far the most common cause of brain injuries; there are nearly 800,000 new strokes in the United States each year. Often stroke is not considered a brain injury so as to avoid confusion with traumatic brain injury or some of the other causes noted above. The strokes which present clinically most like a typical "brain injury" are hemorrhagic strokes and very large strokes, especially if there is edema (swelling) causing increased pressure in the brain. This is because it causes a more global brain impairment. While the initial management of stroke is different in the acute hospital, the rehabilitation period may be similar, especially if there is a lot of cognitive or behavioral impairment resulting from the stroke.

The biggest difference between stroke and a traumatic brain injury is the increased risk of recurrence. The greatest risk factor for a stroke is having had a previous stroke. Therefore, it is very important for a person who has suffered a stroke to take measures to reduce his or her risk of stroke. Previous strokes become a lifelong risk factor so the person who had the stroke should always make every effort to comply with his or her doctor's recommendations to minimize risk factors. See the book, *Managing Stoke: A Guide to Living Well after Stroke,* for more details on stroke in the References section.

KEY POINTS

- The symptoms of nontraumatic brain injury and its rehabilitation can be very similar to TBI so most of the information in this book will apply to anyone who has suffered any type of brain injury.
- The medical management of a nontraumatic brain injury may be different from that of TBI and, therefore, should be discussed with a doctor who is familiar with the person who had the brain injury.

4

BRAIN TUMORS

JENNIFER HENDRICKS

Half of the fight of recovering from a brain tumor is repairing what's broken; half the fight is learning to adapt to what has changed. For example, the tumor weakened the left side of my body and caused left-side neglect. So while my left arm and leg slowly regain strength, I will always have to remind myself to pay attention to the left side of the universe . . . look all the way to the left. —Brendan Ogg

A chapter on brain tumors has been included in this book because the symptoms of a brain tumor, and the rehabilitation process, are sometimes similar to other brain injuries. Also in recent years, increasing numbers of individuals have been admitted following treatment for a brain tumor. However, unlike other acquired brain injuries, in which there is a sudden neurological change caused by the injury followed by recovery, tumors may get gradually worse, even after surgery or rehabilitation. Therefore, this topic is being addressed in its own chapter as some of the information and resources are very different.

There are many different types of brain tumors. Brain tumors can be benign or malignant. Benign tumors do not contain cancer cells. They do not invade tissue around them or spread to other parts of the body. However, they can press on sensitive areas of the brain and cause serious problems. Malignant tumors contain cancer cells. Cancer cells are cells that form when the body does not need them. The cells form a mass of tissue or tumor. They are likely to grow more rapidly than benign tumors and can invade healthy brain tissue.

Tumors that begin in the brain are called primary tumors. Primary brain tumors are named according to the type of cell or the part of brain in which they begin. The tumor is assigned a grade, ranging from grade I to grade IV. Grade I is the least aggressive; the more aggressive the tumor, the higher its grade.

Brain tumors that begin somewhere else in the body are called secondary tumors or metastatic tumors. They are formed by the same type of abnormal cell as the part of the body they come from and have the same name as that type of cancer. For example, lung cancer that spreads to the brain would be described as metastatic lung cancer with "mets" (metastases) to brain, not as "brain cancer." Secondary or metastatic tumors are more common than primary tumors.

Tumors are often found because a person has symptoms suggesting there may be a problem. Symptoms of brain tumors depend on the size, type, and location of the tumor. The symptom may be caused by pressure it is putting on a part of the brain or fluid built up within the skull caused by swelling in the brain. Symptoms can also be caused by a tumor pressing on a nerve. Common symptoms of brain tumors are headaches, nausea, vomiting, and seizures. Other common signs include changes in speech, vision, or hearing; problems with balance or walking; weakness or numbness or tingling in the arms or legs. Changes in mood, personality, memory, or ability to concentrate are also frequently noted. Keep in mind that none of these symptoms are diagnostic of a brain tumor.

When symptoms suggest a brain tumor, the doctor will perform a neurologic exam and likely obtain a CT scan or MRI of the brain. Once the tumor is found, a surgeon may perform a biopsy or take cells from the tumor. The biopsy sample will be sent to a pathologist who determines the type of tumor based on the type of cells in the tumor. There are times when it is not possible to biopsy a tumor. If it is in a part of the brain where the risk of damaging normal brain tissue is too great, the doctor will instead use information obtained from the CT, MRI, or other imaging tests.

Many people decide to talk with more than one doctor about their tumor. There are a number of ways to find a doctor to get a second opinion. The doctor who diagnosed the tumor can often suggest a specialist at another cancer center. Many local, regional, and national community resources can help with finding an appropriate specialist. One such resource is the Cancer Information Service (1-800-4-CANCER). Consultations can be requested with a team of specialists at the Neuro-Oncology Branch of the Warren Grant Magnuson Clinical Center at the National Institutes of Health in Bethesda, Maryland. The American Board of Medical Specialties (ABMS) Directory of Board Certified Medical Specialists may also be of some assistance. ABMS lists names and specialties of physicians who are board certified in a variety of areas. Their phone number is 1-866-ASK-ABMS. For additional information, their website is http://www.abms.org.

COMMON BRAIN TUMORS

As mentioned previously, the most common brain tumors are metastatic brain tumors. However, this section reviews the more common types of primary brain tumors.

Astrocytoma

Astrocytomas are the most common type of glioma. They are formed by star-shaped glial cells called astrocytes, which are supporting cells in the brain. They can occur in most parts of the brain including the brain stem. In children, most astrocytomas are low-grade. In adults, these are usually high-grade tumors. Low-grade astrocytomas tend to grow slowly and are localized to one part of the brain. Higher grade astrocytomas tend to grow quickly and invade surrounding brain tissue. Glioblastoma multiforme (GBM, grade IV astrocytoma) is the most aggressive and most common form of in adults. Anaplastic astrocytroma (grade III) is the second most common form in adults. In adults, the majority of these tumors are in the cerebral hemispheres, which are above the brainstem and cerebellum. In children, however, they more commonly involve the part of the brain that includes the cerebellum and brainstem. Therefore, the symptoms associated with the tumors may be different, even though it is the same type of tumor.

Central Nervous System (CNS) Lymphoma

CNS lymphoma typically appears in the form of brain or spinal cord tumors. The tumor is formed by lymphocyte cells or white blood cells. These cells are a normal part of the body's immune system.

Ependymoma

Ependymoma is a tumor formed by glioma cells from the ependymal cells that line the ventricles of the brain and central canal of the spinal cord.

Medulloblastoma

Medulloblastomas are called primitive neuroectodermal tumors (PNET). PNET tumors arise in the cerebellum and are the most common type of malignant brain tumor in children. However, they also occur in adults. It is usually an aggressive and invasive tumor. It can spread throughout the central nervous system by the spinal fluid.

Meningioma

Meningiomas develop from the meninges, the thin, protective membrane covering the brain and spinal cord. They usually grow slowly and do not invade surrounding brain tissue. The majority of these types of tumor are benign. They are typically single, slow-growing tumors, but some people may have multiple meningiomas and/or meningioms that grow quickly and even recur after surgery.

Oligodendroglioma

This type of brain tumor develops from glial cells called oligodendroglia. These cells form the covering insulation of the nerve fibers within the brain. A tumor formed of only oligodendroglia cells is unusual. More often, they are a mix of astrocyte and oligodendrocyte cells. They may also contain mineral deposits.

Pituitary Tumors

Pituitary tumors are also called adenomas. The term adenoma is used for tumors that arise from gland cells; it is not specific for tumors of the pituitary gland. Here, however, we are referring to tumors that are formed in the pituitary gland, a small oval shaped structure located at the base of the brain. This gland releases hormones that help control the body's other glands and influence the body's growth and metabolism. This type of tumor is usually benign.

Schwannomas

Vestibular schwannomas are also known as acoustic neuromas. This type of tumor tends to be slow-growing and benign. It is a tumor of the 8th cranial nerve, which contains nerve cells important for hearing and balance.

TREATMENT OF BRAIN TUMORS

The recommended treatment of brain tumors is based on the type, location, size, and grade of the tumor(s). Tumors are treated with surgery, radiation, and/or chemotherapy. Surgery is often recommended for brain tumors, particularly if the tumor itself is causing symptoms due to pressure on the brain. During surgery, the skull is opened; this procedure is called a craniotomy. After surgeons remove all or part of the tumor, they cover the opening with the part of skull they removed or with a piece of metal or fabric. Sometimes surgery is not possible or recommended. The surgeon may not be able to remove the tumor without damaging normal brain tissue. Radiation therapy may be suggested instead. Radiation uses high-energy rays to kill tumor cells. The radiation comes from x-rays, gamma rays, or protons. A large machine aims a beam of radiation at the tumor. The type of radiation treatment depends on the type, size, and location of the tumor. Chemotherapy is also used to kill tumor cells. Some individuals receive a combination of these treatments. Following is a list of questions that may be helpful to ask the doctor or other members of the treatment team before starting treatment:

- What type of brain tumor is it?
- Is it benign or malignant?
- What is the grade of the tumor?
- What type of treatment is generally recommended for my type of tumor?
- What are the benefits and risks of treatment?
- Is the treatment covered by my insurance?
- How will the treatment affect my normal activities?
- Should I participate in a clinical trial or research study that treats the specific tumor I have?

It is often helpful to have another person present in addition to the patient at the medical appointments. That way both the patient and caregivers can ask the questions and the caregiver can write down the doctor's responses. The patient can therefore concentrate on what the doctor is saying. The questions and answers can be overwhelming. Writing down the information can help one to remember what was discussed.

Treatments and Therapies

At any stage of treatment someone with a brain tumor, or those around him, may notice symptoms that are affecting daily function or quality of life. These symptoms should be brought to the attention of the doctor who may suggest care for such symptoms. Some treatments are focused on controlling pain or other symptoms caused by the tumor itself, whereas other treatments are to relieve side effects of the radiation or chemotherapy, or to ease the emotional effects of the situation.

A variety of procedures and medications support people with brain tumors. Some types will help with side effects of the tumor or treatment while others are intended to slow the progression of the tumor.

Steroids help relieve swelling of the brain. Steroids are usually started before the surgery if there is significant swelling around the tumor. They are also used in the initial period after the procedure as well. The dose is usually high to start to decrease swelling as quickly as possible and then gradually tapered to avoid the many potential side effects of remaining on a course of steroids for a long time. Steroids, whether for long-term or short-term use, have the potential for causing many side effects. The patient should discuss these with the doctor.

Brain tumors can cause seizures. Anticonvulsants may be recommended to prevent or control seizures. For more information on these and other medications, see Chapter 8 on medications.

A shunt is a tube placed in the brain to allow excess fluid to drain outside the body or into the abdominal cavity (ventriculo-peritoneal shunt or VP shunt). Shunts and drains are used if too much cerebrospinal fluid (CSF) is accumulating in the ventricles, a condition called hydrocephalus. The ventricles are a fluid-filled space containing CSF. However, too much fluid can result in unwanted neurological changes. A shunt may be placed to drain the fluid, reversing or improving the neurological symptoms.

Palliative care focuses on the relief of pain and other symptoms. It can help individuals to regain the strength to carry on with their daily lives. This type of care is appropriate at any time during a serious illness. It is not based on prognosis for recovery. Palliative care can be provided at the same time as curative or life-extending treatment. Palliative care is usually provided by healthcare teams specializing in this kind of care. The team may include doctors, nurses, social workers, chaplains, psychologists, massage therapists, pharmacists, and dietitians. The team works in partnership with the primary care doctor.

Complementary and alternative medicine is a growing area of healthcare that focuses on using nontraditional treatments, for example nutritional supplements, herbal medicines, and acupuncture. Many individuals use complementary and alternative medicine to decrease the negative effects of treatment or decrease symptoms related to the tumor. Unfortunately, people who use these alternative treatments often neglect to tell their physicians about it because they may not consider it "medicine." However, it is very important to tell all treating doctors so they can work effectively with the entire treatment team and effectively evaluate symptoms and responses to therapy. Furthermore, some of the treatments, although safe by themselves, may have potential interactions with chemotherapy, radiation therapy, and/or other treatments being prescribed. For these reasons, it is necessary for all treating physicians to know everything that their patients are using in their treatment to ensure they are providing the best care.

Rehabilitation may be needed if the tumor or treatment has affected activities of daily living, thinking, behavior, or communication. Tumors can cause weakness and problems with balance. Physical therapy can help to regain strength and balance. Occupational therapy helps to manage activities, such as eating, using the bathroom, bathing, and dressing. Speech therapy can help with speaking, expressing thoughts, thinking or memory, or swallowing. Neuropsychology, along with the other types of therapy provided in rehabilitation, can assist with various aspects of thinking, memory, and problem solving. Psychology, social work, and case management will help the person with a tumor and his or her family adapt to and cope with having a brain tumor. These specialists can help to provide the emotional or social supports needed. The goals of rehabilitation are based on a person's mobility, the ability to complete tasks of daily living, and his or her thinking and communication. There may also be goals for higher levels of functioning, such as driving, raising children, and returning to work. The interventions will be focused on building strength, learning new ways of performing tasks, and educating and training the person with impairments and his or her caregivers.

Emotional Support

The emotional impact of a brain tumor in some ways is similar to that of a brain injury. However, there are some aspects of living with a brain tumor that are different. Being given the diagnosis of a brain tumor can be an emotionally traumatic experience for the person with the tumor as well as friends and family. Many people report being shocked when told they have a brain tumor. Unlike a traumatic brain injury in which the struggle is recovery from a single event, having a brain tumor means there may be a need to go through rehabilitation for injury to the brain while the tumor is being treated—and potentially is still growing—thus causing more problems. The impact to the health of a person with a brain tumor is very serious, regardless of whether the tumor is benign or malignant. While much of the treatment is focused on removing and treating the tumor, it is just as important for the team of professionals to focus on helping with emotional adjustment to the situation. Recent studies have found that familial and emotional concern rather than physical concerns tends to be more of a source of stress for long-term survivors of brain tumors. Depression and anxiety have also been strongly correlated with quality of life. Therefore, it is critical to have an increase in awareness of the source and level of stress so that interventions are started, when necessary, to decrease distress and improve quality of life.

Caregivers

A caregiver's distress may be related to an increase in the burden of caring for a loved one. Research has found that a decrease in perceived burden can mean a decrease in distress for the caregiver. Assisting the person with a brain tumor with toileting, dressing, and walking can be very difficult. Friends and extended family members may be able to assist with transportation, cooking, and laundry. However, it is more challenging for extended family or friends to assist with more intimate levels of caregiving. It is important for the treatment team to focus their training with caregivers. The caregiver needs to know what symptoms the person may experience and how to deal with them. Behavioral and emotional changes are sometimes the most difficult for a caregiver to face. The primary caregiver may need counseling and extra emotional support to help cope with this situation. It is as important for caregivers to have sounding boards and people with whom they can talk about the situation as it is for the person with the tumor. The stress associated with the change in roles within the family should not be underestimated. Recognition of family role changes and the psychosocial effects on the caregiver can be critical in taking care of the patient and their loved ones. To put it simply, caregivers need care as well. For more information and resources available for persons with brain tumors, see Appendix D.

KEY POINTS

- Brain tumors include primary brain tumors and metastatic tumors. The primary tumors may be malignant (cancerous) or nonmalignant, but all tumors can cause neurologic symptoms.
- Treatment of brain tumors includes surgery, chemotherapy, and radiation therapy.
- Palliative care is treatment of the symptoms to improve quality of life.

—5—
PHYSICAL EFFECTS OF BRAIN INJURY

ALISON CUNEO
KELLY PETERSON
OLIVIA GLOVER

*My therapists helped me understand that people who sustain
traumatic brain injury have to re-establish pathways from
the brain to the body. In order to do this, they have to learn
everything all over again. I had to relearn how to walk,
relearn how to talk, relearn how to concentrate and read, relearn
how to perform daily activities.* —Rabbi Lynne Landsberg

Physical changes are often the most
obvious initial result of brain injury as cognitive and behavioral changes
may be difficult to see with one's eyes. Many physical changes can take
place after brain injury. These changes can vary greatly and depend on
what part of the brain was injured and to what extent. It is unusual for
a person with a moderate to severe brain injury to have only one type of
impairment, for example, having only weakness or just sensory loss.
More often, people present with many impairments after brain injury,
such as weakness and sensory loss on one side of the body, visual
changes, and trouble with balance. If there is more isolated physical
impairment, it could be related to direct trauma to a muscle or nerve in
a limb rather than injury to the brain itself.

Because of differences in the exact location or severity of a brain
injury, the physical changes may be different for any two people who
suffered what appeared to be similar brain injuries. In most cases, the
brain controls the opposite side of the body. For example, if a person
injures the right side of the brain, he or she may have difficulty moving

the left side of the body. It is important to take into consideration that it can be difficult to determine how someone will recover because of the variability of brain injuries. Nonetheless, while it may not be possible to predict the final outcome, the therapists can still help preserve function in the very early period and later to facilitate regaining motor control as the brain heals in order to maximize functional recovery. It is important to remember that the brain takes time to heal, so it will take time to regain function.

EARLY CHANGES

In the early period after a brain injury, a person may have trouble with regulating normal bodily functions. The patient may grind his or her teeth, sweat profusely, have an elevated heart rate or temperature, or have altered breathing patterns. These are signs of a hyperadrenergic state, a common condition after brain injury. Although these are usually abnormal signs in a healthy person, a person who has sustained a brain injury may exhibit these signs as the brain heals. In addition, one may experience changes in blood pressure especially when changing positions such as sitting up in bed. The use of compression stockings or an elastic binder on the abdomen can help to maintain blood pressure levels. During the time of these early physical changes, it is important to monitor these bodily functions and prevent any secondary complications as they may limit the person's ability to tolerate and benefit from therapy.

Another important complication that may occur early or late in the recovery process is skin breakdown (pressure ulcers or decubitus ulcers). These ulcers can result from decreased sensation or the inability to move independently. Therefore, monitoring for early skin changes and preventing pressure ulcers is imperative.

Initially, a person recovering from a brain injury can have a decreased level of consciousness or arousal. He or she may show a decreased ability to respond to various stimuli, including loud noises and pain, and may show very little voluntary movement. After a severe brain injury, some characteristic postures can lead to complications if not appropriately addressed through rehabilitation. Decorticate posturing is when a person's arms bend (flex) and the legs extend, and decerebrate posturing is when all extremities extend. These postures can lead to skin breakdown as well as joint contractures if not adequately addressed. These abnormal postures tend to diminish as the person begins to regain normal movement.

Even before the person is responding, he or she will begin to have therapy. Daily exercises will be performed by the therapists. Therapists can show the caregivers how to help with these exercises. The person with a brain injury may demonstrate movement; however, it may be nonpurposeful. Restlessness, as demonstrated by the person rolling around in bed, kicking, or waving his or her arms, teeth-grinding, or head turning, are also very common. This type of movement seen with restlessness can sometimes cause safety concerns, placing the person at risk of falling or accidental trauma to the limbs.

Caregivers can alert medical staff of changes observed in the brain-injured person's physical appearance while visiting. Caregivers can also assist to reposition him or her by laying the patient on his or her side and moving the arms and legs carefully through range-of-motion exercises, which will help decrease stiffness. However, before assisting in any exercises, caregivers should receive training on how to perform these tasks safely.

MOVEMENT CHANGES

There can be a variety of motor presentations in persons after traumatic brain injury. Although the muscles may not have been directly injured, often the connections between the brain and the muscles have been damaged. Sometimes the person with brain injury will have weakness or difficulty controlling his or her movements. One may also see weakness on one side of the body; this is called hemiplegia (complete or nearly complete paralysis) or hemiparesis (weakness). Usually weakness presents on the side of the body opposite to the side of the brain that was injured. For example, an injury to the left side of the brain may cause deficits on the right side of the body. Sometimes, however, because of more widespread injury or a mass effect putting pressure on the opposite side of the brain, the weakness may not be limited to just the opposite side of the body.

Weakness on one side of the body can often cause problems with muscle imbalance as the stronger side tries to overpower the weaker side. Hemiplegia can affect both a person's arm and leg to the same extent or can be more pronounced in one compared to the other. Additionally, depending on which parts of the brain are affected, the injury may cause certain muscle groups to be weaker than others. For example, muscles that flex the arm at the elbow may be stronger than ones that straighten the arm. The most common pattern after a stroke or brain injury is the arm will be flexed and the leg will be extended. This muscle imbalance can lead to contractures or functional problems that the therapists can target in rehabilitation. People with brain injury may regain large movements sooner but may not have the small, coordinated movements to complete tasks such as buttoning a shirt or writing their name. Caregivers can assist by observing the person's posture in bed and in the wheelchair to see if it is in straight alignment. If the patient is leaning more toward one side or looks uncomfortable, the caregiver can ask for assistance to reposition him or her to ensure midline orientation (sitting straight in the chair). Therapists can also teach caregivers certain exercises to perform with the person with a brain injury to supplement the therapy.

Muscle tone is the amount of tension or resistance in a muscle at rest. One needs a certain amount of tone for normal posture and body support. The typical course of change in muscle tone after a brain injury is progression from flaccid (no muscle activity) to spastic (too much muscle activity) to normal tone. Right after an injury, a person's body or body segments may be flaccid or limp, which means there is no movement present. The person's limbs will feel heavy at this point and may also show some swelling. Caregivers can assist by handling or moving the person's flaccid or limp body part carefully as the joints may be unstable. Further injury could happen with aggressive movement. Persons with brain injury are also often encouraged to elevate their weaker side on pillows to decrease swelling and protect their arms or legs. It is very important to handle these limbs carefully, especially a flaccid arm, as injury can be caused at the shoulder if someone pulls on a flaccid arm. A flaccid arm should always be supported, either on a lap tray in a wheelchair or using a sling, to prevent the shoulder from subluxing (coming out of the socket).

WHAT IS SPASTICITY?

Often the next stage is spastic movement. Spasticity is increased muscle tone caused by impairment in the brain's ability to inhibit (stop or control) the firing of nerves. The muscles are working more as a reflex. It is at this stage especially that daily stretching and range of motion (ROM) exercises must be completed. Because these spastic muscles can overcome the weaker ones, it is important to keep the joints moving in all directions, even if the muscles are not strong enough to move them yet. Spasticity can lead to stiffness, and sometimes contractures. A joint contracture is when a joint becomes "frozen" in one position and the limb at that joint cannot be moved. Spasticity and/or poor positioning can contribute to the development of contractures. Often, as contractures are just starting to evolve, they can be treated with stretching, prolonged weight-bearing, and sometimes with splinting or casting over a period of time to stretch out the shortened muscles. It is very common for therapists to prescribe splints or casts to maintain good joint alignment for persons after brain injury. Although the materials used are similar to those used for orthopedic injuries, they are not used for the same purpose. However, when conservative methods have failed, surgery can be considered to lengthen the tendons. Every effort is made to avoid surgery. In addition to the therapies discussed above, medications can be used to help decrease spasticity as well. (See Chapter 8.)

The ultimate goal is getting back to normal movement patterns. Although some people do achieve this, they still may experience some involuntary movements during stressful situations or when they are completing a very challenging movement. For example, a person with a brain injury may show normal muscle tone when sitting, but the arm may begin to bend when he or she is walking or climbing stairs.

MOTOR CONTROL

The ability to control movement is also often impaired after a brain injury. A person may have good strength, but may be unable to control the movement to perform physical functions.

Apraxia is the inability to perform a task despite the strength to do so. It is an inability of the brain to send the proper signal to make the body function as desired. Apraxia can be difficult to explain and presents itself in ways that seem very unusual. In some cases, people are unable to imitate a motor task or gesture despite fully understanding the idea or concept of the task. In other cases, people may inappropriately use tools to perform tasks. For example, someone may use a toothbrush to comb his hair or a spoon to brush his teeth. Apraxia can also be seen when a person dresses as he places the wrong body part in clothing, such as putting his arm through a pant leg. Frequently, having the therapist guide the movements and using repetition will assist people in relearning the appropriate ways to complete these functional tasks.

Ataxia is a term to describe the lack of coordinated movement. It can occur in the trunk and head or in the limbs. Ataxia often leads to problems with balance and the inability to catch oneself before falling. Additionally, ataxia can cause difficulty in reaching for, or holding onto, items. Sometimes people need additional stability to act in a more coordinated way. For example, a person may need to prop his or her elbows on a table to feed himself or herself or wear weighted cuffs to help stabilize a limb.

The overall motor functioning after brain injury is quite complex. Ask the therapists about specific hints for handling or moving a person after a brain injury.

SENSORY CHANGES

Sensory problems include difficulties feeling light touch, pressure, temperature changes, pain, vibration, or recognizing where a limb is in space (without looking). Decreased sensation can limit a person's ability to use the body successfully as he or she may not be able to sense all parts of it. Sensory deficits can cause significant safety issues. For instance, if someone touches a hot plate, the normal reaction is to withdraw the hand to avoid being burned; but if the person does not feel the heat, he or she may get burned. Another sensory deficit that is often present is the lack of feeling where one's body is in space. Proprioception is the ability to know where one's limb or body is in space without visualizing it. Impaired proprioception can lead to functional difficulty and injury. For example, if the person cannot feel his or her ankle rolling over when he or she is standing on it, one may end up with an ankle sprain, but may not even be able to feel or recognize it. If this person cannot feel where his or her body parts are, he or she may also have to look at an object when reaching for it or holding it so that it does not drop on the floor.

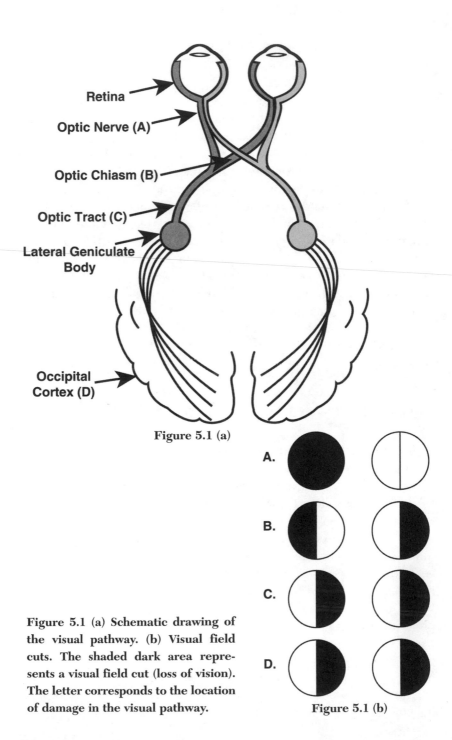

Figure 5.1 (a)

A.

B.

C.

D.

Figure 5.1 (a) Schematic drawing of the visual pathway. (b) Visual field cuts. The shaded dark area represents a visual field cut (loss of vision). The letter corresponds to the location of damage in the visual pathway.

Figure 5.1 (b)

VISUAL AND PERCEPTUAL CHANGES

Visual and perceptual deficits are sensory deficits that occur frequently and can cause some of the most profound impairments. It is common for these problems to persist long after rehabilitation is over, and often they are permanent. There may be an injury to the eyes themselves or to the visual pathways in the brain. Visual deficits can include acuity changes, double vision, decreased eye movements, visual field loss, visual inattention, neglect, and visual processing difficulties. A person with a brain injury may report difficulty seeing but be unable to explain exactly what he or she is experiencing. He or she may show very little or no attention to one side of his or her environment, keeping the head always turned to the opposite side. This may be caused by a visual field cut or a perceptual deficit. One common presentation is when vision is lost in one half (e.g., left only) of both of the eyes, which is called a homonymous hemianopsia. Figure 5.1 is a diagram showing homonymous hemianopsia. The dark area is the part of the visual field that is lost.

A person with a brain injury may neglect one side of his or her body or environment. In this case, caregivers can assist by placing things of interest on the neglected side and talk to the person from this side to encourage head turning and attention to that side.

Double vision, or diplopia, is another visual deficit that is commonly seen. The person may cover up one eye when looking at something to accommodate for this deficit.

Visual perceptual deficits may hinder a person's ability to complete many other functional tasks because the perception and understanding of physical or cognitive tasks may be limited. A person with a brain injury may be evaluated by a neuro-ophthalmologist who will be able to provide a thorough assessment of the patient's visual difficulties.

FATIGUE

Fatigue often sets in much earlier in a patient than prior to the injury. A person's endurance drastically decreases after being in the hospital for even a few days. Activities that may have previously been done easily, such as getting dressed, may now require much of a person's energy.

Initially a person may only be able to tolerate an activity for a few minutes before needing a rest break. Incorporating rest breaks will be important for maximizing recovery. Energy conservation strategies, such as spacing out taxing activities or completing activities in a seated position, may help the person with a brain injury to become more independent. Cognitive fatigue may also be contributing to feelings of exhaustion as the patient is being asked to concentrate and learn new things daily.

BLADDER AND BOWEL CONTROL

Following brain injury, people can have difficulty managing bodily functions including bladder and bowel control. This difficulty may be caused by several factors. Often the message from the brain does not travel to the bladder or bowel as efficiently as it did before the brain injury and can result in incontinence or retention. This situation is referred to as a neurogenic bladder or neurogenic bowel. Incontinence is uncontrolled emptying of urine at an unplanned time or location. Urinary retention occurs when the bladder holds too much urine and becomes over-stretched. Dribbling can occur because of overflow. The retained urine in the bladder can also contribute to an increased likelihood of infection. Another problem can be an overactive bladder. This problem is a result of overactive nerves controlling the bladder and causing bladder "spasms." This kind of incontinence can occur during sleep, after drinking water, or when listening to running water. Additionally, people with brain injuries may have difficulty standing or sitting because of weakness that limits the ability to sit on a toilet to urinate. An upright position for toileting causes increased abdominal pressure that aides the process. Toileting while lying in bed using a bedpan or urinal can be more difficult.

Continence is also a cognitive skill since the subtle signs that a person needs to use the toilet must be recognized. When a person is unable to recognize the need to go to the toilet, where the toilet is, or get to the toilet in time, incontinence can become an issue. Causes of incontinence in this case can be confusion, poor eyesight, unwillingness to toilet because of depression, anxiety, anger, or physical limitations making it difficult to reach the toilet in time. Interventions that may be used for incontinence include toileting schedules, use of bedside commodes, medications, catheterizations, bladder scans, and incontinence products. Caregivers can assist with bladder control by asking the rehabilitation team what intervention is being used and encouraging consistency.

SKIN AND WOUND CARE

Some commonly heard terms regarding skin following brain injury are abrasions (caused by friction) and lacerations (made by cutting). It is common for persons who have been in traumatic accidents to have abrasions or lacerations on their bodies. The person or caregiver may also notice increased sweating and worsening of acne as well as rashes and other skin conditions, which can be caused by medication reactions or a reaction to tape, detergents, or other products used in the hospital.

As a complication of prolonged bed rest or immobility caused by brain injury, one may get a pressure sore. A pressure sore is an injury to the skin and/or underlying tissue usually over a bony prominence as a result of pressure, or pressure in combination with shearing or friction. Caregivers should be aware of several contributing factors and risk factors in regards to pressure ulcers, including moisture, immobility/inactivity, poor nutrition/hydration, decreased blood flow, and medical comorbidities, such as diabetes, respiratory failure, and obesity.

Caregivers should also be aware that bony prominences are possible risk areas for sores. Hips, coccyx, buttocks, heels, elbows, shoulder blades, and back of the head are risk areas. The sores on the buttocks may be a result of lying in bed for prolonged periods which typically causes sacral ulcers (over the sacral bone). Sores that occur as a result of sitting in a chair for long periods of time are usually ischial ulcers (over the ischial bones). Sores are generally seen on the lower half of the body. Pressure may also be noticed along the edges of casts and splints. Pressure sores are the most common complication of physical disability or chronic illness. Three percent to sixty-six percent of all hospitalized persons develop a pressure sore during their hospital stay. The risk of developing a pressure ulcer is greater for people who had prolonged ICU stays, have impaired sensation and are not able to turn themselves in bed. Also, incontinence is a risk factor as the moisture places the skin at increased risk for breakdown.

There are many ways to prevent skin breakdown. Members of the person's care team as well as family and caregivers can monitor and encourage frequent position changes when in bed and seated in a chair as well as proper transfer and bed mobility techniques. It is also very important to maintain dry, moisturized skin, ensure frequent skin checks, provide adequate nutrition and hydration, and maintain communication with the team if skin changes are noticed.

ORTHOPEDIC CONCERNS

Often, if the brain injury was caused by an accident of some kind, the person may also have orthopedic injuries as well as a brain injury. These injuries may include sprains, strains, or broken bones. These injuries will also be addressed in therapy and may produce additional difficulties, such as an inability to put weight through a broken limb. If a the doctor advises the patient to remain nonweight-bearing to allow a bone to heal, the therapists will teach him or her alternative ways to complete his or her activities of daily living and mobility. It is very important, however, that the patient and his or her caregivers adhere to the weight-bearing precautions and other orthopedic restrictions so that fractured bones may heal properly. Although most orthopedic injuries are diagnosed and treated in the acute hospital, a person with a brain injury may not be able to communicate, thereby limiting the initial evaluation. Therefore, if a person with a brain injury begins to have "new" pain during rehabilitation, it does not necessarily imply a new injury. Rather, it may indicate an improved ability to communicate about symptoms, such as pain, from an injury that occurred at the time of the accident. This finding should be reported to the rehabilitation team so it can be evaluated appropriately.

In addition to the orthopedic injuries, nerve injuries that occur in the arms or legs (peripheral nerve injuries) can result from direct trauma to the limb. Therefore, it is important to remember that not all weakness or pain is directly related to the brain injury. If there is pain, weakness or sensory changes that do not correlate to the lesion in the brain or those that do not improve at the same rate as everything else, it is possible that there has also been a peripheral nerve injury.

WHAT TO EXPECT FROM THERAPY

Physical changes will affect people in many ways and may limit independence. Therapists will address these deficits as they relate to functional activities with a goal of increased independence in mind. Functional activities that may be addressed in therapy include bathing, dressing, walking, toileting, feeding, positioning in bed, climbing stairs, eating, propelling a wheelchair, and participating in household tasks like cooking and cleaning. There are many physical building blocks required to achieve independence in these tasks, which will be addressed in therapy.

Therapy in Union

Cognition and behavior can play a big part in physical recovery as well. Sometimes, a person may be able to move around in bed unaided, yet will be unable to follow a command to move. He or she may be able to walk without assistance but be unable to find the bathroom. In this case, all therapies come together to work on common goals to such as overall independence and safety.

CAREGIVER'S ROLE IN THE REHABILITATION PROCESS

As addressed throughout this chapter, the caregiver can be involved in many aspects of care. Caregivers can help by communicating to the therapists the interests of the patient as well as how he or she was func tioning prior to the brain injury. Caregivers can also help by participating in therapy sessions with the therapists and medical staff to learn how to assist in a manner that is safe to both the person with the brain injury and the caregiver himself. Caregiver training is of utmost importance prior to discharge to ensure the safety of the person with a brain injury as well as the caregiver. Depending on the severity of the brain injury, a person may require a caregiver for months or years after the injury. Many of the issues discussed in this chapter will be long-term problems that a person with a brain injury will face. He or she will need the caregiver to provide the best possible care and "maintenance" therapy at home to minimize any complications.

KEY POINTS

- There are many changes that can occur after brain injury, including:
  - Motor difficulties, including trouble with motor control, motor planning, and tone
  - Sensory deficits, including vision and perception
  - Fatigue
  - Bladder and bowel control
  - Skin integrity
  - Orthopedic issues
- All persons with brain injury in rehabilitation will receive therapy to address their specific needs in preparation for a safe discharge.
- Caregivers play a major role throughout the rehab process. It is important for all caregivers to be involved in the care of the person with a brain injury during all phases of rehabilitation.

6

COGNITIVE AND COMMUNICATION EFFECTS OF BRAIN INJURY

INBAL ESCHEL
BROWNRIGG SNOW

[Fred] was beginning to make his way back, but it was the music of [his] favorite Motown group that really seemed to make a real difference in his recovery. A therapist recommended that I bring in CDs for Fred to listen to as a way to help improve his communication skills. So, I flooded his room with the Temptations music and sang along. Pretty soon, Fred was joining in. He was singing "My Girl" before he really started talking very much. —Sharon Douglas

The brain is our control center. It controls all of our actions and feelings, which can include any movement, emotions, and thinking. You will learn more about the physical and emotional changes after brain injury in other chapters of this book. The following sections will focus on the cognitive and communicative changes that can happen after an acquired brain injury.

As discussed in the chapters regarding the brain and its functions, different parts of the brain control different functions. The changes seen after a brain injury depend upon the areas of the brain that were injured. The injury, and how it affects various cognitive and communicative functions, may range from mild to profound. Although each brain is similar in many ways, we are all unique. Brain injury in the same region of the brain may impact different people in different ways. Also, a child's brain is considered more "flexible" than those of adults and might recover better or faster than adults with similar damage. A person's rate and degree of progress are also impacted by the severity of the injury, preinjury abilities, motivation, and support.

With a moderate to severe injury, swelling in the brain may cause pressure on a lower part of the brain, called the brainstem, which controls consciousness. Many people who suffer these types of injuries are in an unconscious state called a coma. There are different levels of consciousness, one of which may involve being unresponsive to any type of stimulation. Other levels may involve the ability to move, respond to pain, track the movements of other people, but still be unaware of their surroundings. At these points, communication is usually not possible. Some people recover from a coma and regain the ability to become alert, to communicate, and to participate in rehabilitation.

The effects of a brain injury are usually most pronounced right after the injury, but it is difficult to predict the extent of difficulties that may persist. Problems in the areas of cognition and communication can be devastating and may have a large impact on a person's ability to function effectively in the hospital, home, and community. Along with the natural healing of the brain, rehabilitation will help the person with brain injury and his caregivers to use strategies to compensate for areas of the brain that were damaged. It is very important to be optimistic about recovery and about the future. The injured person and his or her caregivers should learn as much as possible about the changes that have occurred since the traumatic brain injury (TBI) and work closely with rehabilitation specialists to maximize progress throughout the recovery process. Caregivers are critical members of the rehabilitation team.

WHAT DOES IT ALL MEAN?

Cognitive skills are often called "thinking skills," and include attention, orientation, memory, problem-solving, judgment, safety awareness, processing, and awareness of problem areas. We will discuss all of these areas and describe what the caregivers can do to help. Cognitive skills are closely linked with communication skills, including listening and understanding, expressing thoughts and ideas, reading, and writing. Communication skills also include using language socially and understanding the context in which an exchange occurs. Often, together, these are called cognitive-communication skills, and if difficulties arise, they are called cognitive-communication impairments. The exact pattern of problems is different for every person. Information as to how these problems are assessed and treated is discussed later in this chapter.

COGNITIVE IMPAIRMENTS

One of the first stages of recovery in conscious people involves orientation. Orientation includes being aware of oneself (e.g., name), the date (e.g., year), current location (e.g., in the hospital), and the reason for being in that location. These skills may return naturally, but the brain-injured survivor may also need some help. The caregivers can help by making sure a calendar is posted and reviewing it with the person frequently. A memory log can also help. A memory log is a book where this information (e.g., names of family members, phone numbers, appointment, etc.) is written. The caregiver may also want to post labeled pictures of family members and friends in a place where the person with brain injury would be likely to see them. Please note that too many cards or pictures may be overstimulating. The rehabilitation team will help to ensure a proper balance.

Another area that may be impacted by a brain injury is attention. There are three major categories of attention: sustained, selective, and divided. Sustained attention is the ability to focus on one thing over a period of time (e.g., reading a book). Selective attention is the ability to focus on one thing in the presence of distractions (e.g., reading a book in a noisy room). Divided attention, also known as multitasking, is the ability to complete multiple activities at the same time (e.g., keeping track of the game score on TV while having a conversation). All three of these may be impacted to various degrees and can affect everything from being able to focus on an important conversation, to being distracted by the smallest noise, to being able to concentrate on reading. The caregivers can help by trying to keep the environment quiet (e.g., turning off TV or music when discussing something important), encouraging the person with a brain injury to do one thing at a time, encouraging pacing (e.g., tell him or her to "slow down"), and by keeping the environment organized.

Memory can also be affected by a brain injury. Changes in memory can significantly influence how one relates to the world. Most people can remember information they knew well before the injury (long-term memory), but have trouble remembering and learning new information (short-term memory). For example, after a brain injury the injured person may have a hard time remembering what happened earlier in the day, the names of therapists, techniques learned in therapy, or even a conversation that he or she is in the middle of having. The patient may repeat the same questions many times. These are all normal characteristics of a brain injury and the caregivers can help by using the memory logbook, helping him or her to use the daily schedule or a daily planner, keeping a journal or taking notes about daily activities, making to-do lists and helping by crossing off items as they are completed. Always allow for extra time to learn new things. Maintaining routine is also important when helping a person with brain injury deal with short-term memory problems.

In order to get through the day, all people rely on executive functions, which can be thought of as the CEO, or "coach," of the brain. This specifically refers to one's ability to plan, organize, complete, and evaluate activities that we encounter. We use these to complete all tasks, including anything from getting ready in the morning (e.g., first planning what to wear or what to eat for breakfast, then completing these activities, and modifying if anything goes wrong). Problems with executive functions can significantly impact the ability to complete daily living tasks effectively. The caregivers can help by keeping daily routines simple, using the memory book, and sticking with scheduled tasks, breaking activities down into smaller steps, and using checklists to help organize activities (e.g., getting dressed).

Another component of executive functions is problem-solving/reasoning. Each and every day we encounter situations which require thinking through problems and making decisions about how to solve them. An example could be reaching a broken elevator and deciding to take the escalator instead. Typically, we make these decisions subconsciously, or without being truly aware of how we go about it. After a brain injury, it can be more difficult to solve problems and make sound and safe decisions. The person with a brain injury may make decisions quickly, without allowing the time to think through the problem or the consequences. He or she may also try to solve problems in ways that do not make sense. For example, a patient may not think that he or she needs help getting out of bed and to the bathroom so he or she may do this without calling for assistance. That decision is not a safe solution to the problem because of the risk of falling and hurting oneself. Problem-solving requires the ability to decide what the problem is, brainstorm ways to solve it, choose the best and safest decision, and implement it. Caregivers can help break problems down into small, more manageable steps, talk through problems together, and encourage the person to ask for help when needed.

After a brain injury it may take someone more time to think and respond to what's going on in his or her environment. This can be referred to as "processing" information. It may take longer to answer questions and understand what one hears or reads. The caregivers can help by encouraging the patient to ask others to slow down and repeat information as needed. The caregiver or communication partner can also allow for more time to respond, limit the amount of information given at one time, remove distractions from the environment, and give directions one step at a time. To help the person with a brain injury process written material, the caregiver and therapists can assist by writing information of shorter length, encouraging the patient to underline or highlight important information and again allow extra time to process the material.

COMMUNICATION IMPAIRMENTS

Communication can also be impacted by brain injury. Although a person with a brain injury may not have difficulty with finding words and creating sentences to express what he or she is thinking and feeling, there may still be subtle, but critical, communication disruptions. Problems with communication after brain injury often result from problems in various cognitive areas, including attention, memory, organization, problem-solving, and reasoning. Difficulties may include being tangential or off topic, disorganized while talking, having trouble understanding jokes or proverbs, following conversation, paying attention to detail, or making social judgments, including using and understanding facial expression and body language. The concept of making appropriate social judgments also includes taking turns in conversation (e.g., not just talking about oneself, but asking the conversation partner questions as well) and making appropriate eye contact (e.g., looking at the conversation partner during conversation). If the brain injury is more localized on the left side of the brain, the person may experience a language disorder called aphasia.

The ability to stay on topic and be organized in expressing thoughts and ideas may be impacted by brain injury. It may be harder for the person to "get to the point." For example, the patient may be talking about the latest sports game with the caregivers, and all of a sudden, start discussing the weather when it is not related. The caregivers can help by reminding him or her of the topic at hand. A person with a brain injury may have more difficulty understanding "abstract" information, like jokes, proverbs (e.g., "Don't cry over spilled milk"), or sarcasm. Caregivers can help by being more concrete in how they speak (e.g., fewer proverbs, idioms, etc.) and by not expecting a change in facial expression when someone makes a joke. It may also be difficult for the person with a brain injury to make inferences, which are connections between things that are not directly stated, both in conversation and while reading. For example, if the caregiver says, "It's hot in here," a person with a brain injury would not think to turn on the air conditioner. It may be difficult for him or her to follow a conversation because it may be hard (and take longer) to keep track of, and remember, what he or she hears. Caregivers can help by repeating and rephrasing what they said and by asking questions during conversation to make sure that he or she is following along. They can also encourage the patient to repeat the caregivers' statements in his or her own words to make sure he or she understands and remembers it. It is also common for persons with brain injury to demonstrate other difficulties in making good social judgments. For example, after an injury, a person may tell strangers intimate feelings, ask inappropriate personal questions, or make sexual comments. The caregivers can help by calmly letting the person know when he or she is making inappropriate statements, coming up with a system to let him or her know when behavior is inappropriate, and giving positive and negative reinforcement. Please see Behavioral and Emotional Effects of Brain Injury (Chapter 6) for additional information on similar areas.

Aphasia is a language disorder with a range of types and severities. In general, when a person has an aphasia, one can expect difficulties in the following areas: expressing thoughts and ideas verbally, understanding what is being said out loud, understanding what is being read, and expressing thoughts and ideas in writing. Communicating with those who have aphasia can be challenging. The speech-language pathologist

(SLP), also referred to as a speech therapist, will help both the person with a brain injury and the caregivers with communication. Giving the affected persons extra time to express their thoughts and resisting the temptation to speak for them is extremely important. A patient may benefit from the use of a picture or written communication board often provided by the SLP. It may also help to ask questions with yes or no answers rather than "open-ended" questions requiring more speech output. When speaking to someone with aphasia, keep in mind that he or she may not process everything said by the communicating partner. It is important to speak slowly (but naturally), keep statements simple and concrete, give one direction at a time, and remove background noise. Also, only one person should speak at a time. The patient's ability to regain skills or compensate for impairments in reading and writing will be addressed by the SLP.

Assessment/Evaluation

No two individuals are alike, and everyone displays a slightly different pattern of difficulties. The person with a brain injury will need to be evaluated to assess how the rehabilitation team can help. Various members of the rehabilitation team, including the speech-language pathologist, the neuropsychologist, and occupational therapist, will assess the patient's cognitive-communication skills in different ways. The SLP will choose various formal tests to look at the skill areas discussed above, especially the ones with which the person with brain injury is having the most difficulty. In conjunction with the SLP, the neuropsychologist will also initiate formal cognitive testing. Together, the two disciplines can provide a broader picture of the person's impairments and rehabilitation needs. The SLP will also use informal observation (the "trained eye" of the professional) to help determine the patient's strengths and weaknesses. Observation and evaluation from the occupational therapist is another source of input in determining a person's ability to perform activities of daily living (ADLs). For instance, one may have the physical ability to dress and bathe, but have trouble completing the task because of impaired thinking skills. The caregivers can also provide information to help the SLP better understand what the patient's personality and skills were before the brain injury and which characteristics seem to be the most different. The skill areas that seem to need the most help usually form the starting point for creating goals. Part of the evaluation consists of creating short- and long-term goals, which are skills and tools that the SLP will work on with the brain-injured person to help him or her function and communicate as best as possible. Each evaluation is individually tailored. The tests that are used to assess a patient are based on his or her function; not all tests are appropriate for everyone, particularly after a brain injury. In rehabilitation, it is not appropriate to use a standard set of goals for everyone. Both assessment and treatment are based on the individual's needs, requests and input from caregivers, and the treatment team.

Treatment

Based on the results of the evaluation and information from the person with the brain injury and his or her caregivers, the SLP determines which areas need work, then treatment will begin. The overall goal of treatment for cognitive-communication impairment is increasing functional independence, or one's ability to complete everyday tasks more independently, and helping the individual to compensate for changes that have occurred since the brain injury. It is important to note that the goal is not to help him or her improve skills that were not strong before the brain injury; treatment focuses only on the areas that have changed since the brain injury. Just as the evaluation was unique, so is the treatment plan. The person undergoing treatment will be working on specific goals, and the SLP will keep track of progress. The SLP will use different techniques and introduce various strategies to help the patient make progress towards these goals and will most likely train the caregivers.

The earlier treatment begins following the brain injury, the better. Depending on the setting and how much time has passed since the injury, the goals will be formally updated in a new report every week, two weeks, or month (once a week earlier on, then every two weeks, then every month). The SLP will typically see the patient for an hour a day early on, and then less and less frequently. The caregivers will also continue to play a critical role in recovery. The patient will be asked to practice the techniques and strategies learned during his or her speech therapy sessions with caregivers to help maximize the recovery.

One major way in which the SLP helps a patient to function after a brain injury is to teach the affected individual and caregivers compensatory strategies to get around an area of weakness. These compensatory strategies can be used in any number of cognitive-communication areas, including all the ones discussed above.

Often, treatment is provided both individually and in groups. Both of these settings are highly recommended and allow persons with a brain injury to work on the same skills in different ways. In the individual sessions, treatment will focus on different strategies and techniques specific to his or her needs that should help with the cognitive-communication skills that have changed since the brain injury. Groups can be more challenging at times because it can be harder for the patient to pay attention and follow along, but groups do provide a great opportunity to practice the techniques learned in individual sessions. Groups will also allow the patient to see what techniques help other people with similar problems. Groups also give the patient a chance to get to know other people who are going through similar experiences.

Treatment of the person with a brain injury is a process involving teamwork. The occupational therapist is also trained to treat problems in cognition. As mentioned in the assessment section of this chapter, the occupational therapist helps patients to improve their cognitive functioning through daily self-care and home management tasks. The neuropsychologist is another team member who will assist in the treatment of impaired thinking skills. Another role of the neuropsychologist is to help with coping mechanisms to deal with the changes in the patient's life caused by the injury. The neuropsychologist often helps the team and caregivers to deal with any new behavioral concerns which can, in turn, aggravate the cognitive problems. The neuropsychologist also guides the therapists and other team members with ways to best manage possible behavioral and emotional changes. The neuropsychologist may join the therapists in their sessions to best facilitate this process.

SHIFTING GEARS . . .

First we focused on the cognitive-communication impairments that can come from a brain injury. Other areas may be affected as well, including the ability to effectively eat and swallow, along with speaking clearly. We will now focus on these areas.

DYSPHAGIA (SWALLOWING IMPAIRMENTS)

After a brain injury, people may have difficulty swallowing solid foods
and/or liquids. This condition is called dysphagia. Dysphagia can make
it difficult to take in enough food to nourish the body. For some people,
it resolves quickly. For others, it can cause problems that are so severe
that a feeding tube is needed to ensure adequate and healthy food and
nutritional intake. For a person with less severe problems, it can cause
a need to adapt the consistency of food and drink that one is able to eat,
or he or she may need to eat in a certain way. Because eating is such a
critical part of life, it will be one of the very first areas evaluated and
treated (as needed) by your SLP. Most people who have dysphagia right
after a brain injury recover at least some ability to drink and eat safely.
Persons with tracheostomies will also need to be evaluated by an SLP
for their swallowing.

Eating is a complicated process that involves using mouth, tongue,
and throat muscles to chew and swallow food or to drink liquid. These
muscles work together in a coordinated, smooth fashion to help us eat
and drink. Eating and swallowing have three stages: oral, pharyngeal,
and esophageal. First, the food is placed in the mouth, where it is
chewed and mixed with saliva. The food is then moved around by the
tongue, which makes it the right size to swallow. The goal of the first
stage is to prepare the food to be swallowed. The second stage begins
when the tongue pushes the food to the back of the mouth, which trig-
gers a swallowing reflex. The food then moves down the esophagus
toward the stomach. In a normal swallow, without thinking consciously
about it, we close off our windpipe to protect our lungs, preventing food
or liquid from "going down the wrong way." The third stage is when the
food or liquid goes into our esophagus, which carries the food or drink
down into the stomach.

When there is a problem with any of the three stages described
above, one is diagnosed with dysphagia. Some of the problems might
involve weakness in the muscles used for eating and swallowing, like the
tongue, lips, or cheeks, making it difficult to chew, to keep food in the
mouth, or to clear the mouth. Food or liquid may go into the airway
during or after swallowing. This is called aspiration. Other problems
might involve the swallowing reflex or having weak throat muscles that
have trouble moving the food toward the stomach.

People with dysphagia may need to eat a special diet and/or use special strategies to help their swallow work more smoothly. If certain recommendations and techniques are not used, small pieces of food may also go down into the windpipe and then into the lungs (aspiration). This can lead to a lung infection called aspiration pneumonia. In a normal swallow, if food goes into the airway, we cough reflexively to help protect it. After a brain injury, the cough may be weak, or the person's body may not sense that food or liquid has been aspirated, and therefore, will not cough to protect the airway. If the person with dysphagia does not cough when food goes down the airway, it is called silent aspiration. This can be very dangerous because it can lead to aspiration pneumonia, but without any warning signs, such as a cough. If this occured, the SLP would modify the diet and educate the patient and caregivers on techniques for feeding. If dysphagia is severe, the patient may not be able to eat anything by mouth which is usually called NPO (nothing per oral). Typically, feeding tubes, which are placed in the nose or stomach, are temporary and will be removed when the swallow is considered safe for eating by mouth (PO [per oral]).

It is critical that caregivers follow feeding recommendations made by the speech-language pathologist. As noted above, sometimes it is not possible to tell if someone is aspirating without special studies. If the recommendations for feeding are not followed, a person with a brain injury will be at risk for developing an aspiration pneumonia. This pneumonia is a common cause of morbidity since it can cause a significant setback in the recovery process, and it can even cause death.

Dysphagia Evaluation

In most hospitals, the SLP evaluates swallowing disorders after traumatic brain injury. The SLP evaluates not only how well the muscles are working and coordinating for the swallow, but also how the cognitive status of the person with the brain injury is impacting his or her ability to take food by mouth. For example, in the earlier stages of recovery, or in severe brain injury, an individual may be lethargic and have low arousal, which may mean that he or she may not be able to pay attention long enough to eat safely. The person with brain injury may also be agitated and impulsive, and may try to eat too quickly to be safe. The SLP takes all of this information into account and then decides what type of testing is appropriate. One method of assessing the swallow is called a "bedside swallow study," where the SLP observes the person with brain injury while he or she is eating or drinking. The SLP looks for several potential warning signs (including coughing, choking, poor initiation, a wet, gurgly voice, or watery eyes). Another type of assessment is called a "modified barium swallow study," or MBS. In this type of assessment, the SLP and the radiologist watch as the person eats various types of foods on an x-ray video. It allows the SLP and radiologist to objectively evaluate for any problems with the swallow, and to identify exactly what they are and where they are occurring.

For individuals with tracheostomies (trachs), the SLP may use either of the evaluations described above or give what is called a blue dye bedside dysphagia evaluation. The SLP will determine which type of evaluation to conduct based on the status of the trach (e.g., size of trach, toleration of trach plugging, possible use of a speaking valve, and estimated length of the time the trach has been in place). During this evaluation, the SLP works together with the nursing staff. The food or liquid consistency is dyed blue, and the nurse will suction the trach site after the SLP asks the patient to swallow. If the blue dye comes out of the trach site during the suction, the SLP will know that some or all of the food or liquid swallowed went into the airway.

There are two major types of dysphagia: oral and pharyngeal. Oral dysphagia is when there are problems in the mouth, or in the first stage of swallowing (as described above). Pharyngeal dysphagia is when there are problems in the throat. Other problems may occur in the second stage of swallowing (as described above). When there are problems with both of these parts, the condition is called oropharyngeal dysphagia. Just as with the evaluation of cognitive and communication disorders after brain injury, the SLP determines the severity level of the dysphagia and makes treatment recommendations.

Treatment

Treatment of dysphagia after brain injury is done by a certified SLP. Just as each evaluation is individualized, so is the treatment. The SLP will use different techniques and introduce various strategies to help the person with brain injury make progress. The SLP will also train the caregivers who can then help reinforce the strategies learned in treatment. The earlier treatment begins after the brain injury, the better.

Stimulating the muscles used for swallowing may be one area on which the SLP will focus. For example, the person with brain injury may be taught certain exercises for the mouth and tongue. Other exercises may have to do with strengthening certain aspects of the swallow. Compensation techniques may also come into play, in which the person with brain injury is taught new ways to "get around" the swallowing difficulties. For example, the patient may be taught to tuck his or her chin or turn his or her head to one side while swallowing to help compensate for the trouble in swallowing. The caregivers play a critical role in reminding the person with brain injury to use the recommended techniques when eating or drinking. The more practice the person gets in using their strategies, the better.

Another common technique in dysphagia treatment is changing the type and consistency of food and liquid that a person eats. In general, the thicker something is, the easier it is for a person with dysphagia to swallow. For example, applesauce is thicker than water. Thicker foods and drinks take a longer time going through the three stages of the swallow and are, therefore, less likely to get into the windpipe. Thickening liquid, which can be done easily with thickening powder, is one way to make swallowing safer. Some people with brain injury may have a difficult time chewing, and therefore may have an easier time with softer foods. There are various ways to change the consistency of what we eat. For example, foods can be soft, ground, or pureed in a blender to make them easier to chew and swallow. The diet that is easiest to swallow is pureed. A ground diet has slightly more texture than puree, but is still very finely chopped. The next stage is called a soft diet in which the food is almost a regular texture, but without any hard or sticky foods (e.g., steak, rice). The SLP will determine which of the four consistencies of food (puree, ground, soft, or regular) and three consistencies of liquid (nectar thick, honey thick, or thin) is safest for the person with the brain injury and will change the consistency of the diet to accommodate the ongoing needs.

If the primary causes of the dysphagia are cognitive (e.g., limited arousal, attention, etc.), the SLP may defer starting an oral diet until some improvements in those areas occur. He may also start off slowly (e.g., "trials" of the safest consistency of food/liquid) and build up to full meals as the person's swallowing ability and level of arousal improves.

DYSARTHRIA (SPEECH PRODUCTION IMPAIR-MENTS)

Speech is the way we sound when we talk. After a stroke, brain injury, tumor, or other nervous system disease (e.g., Parkinson's disease), the muscles we use for speech can be affected. Dysarthria is a speech disorder that is characterized by weakness, slowness, or uncoordinated movements of muscles we use for speech. Some of those muscles include the tongue, lips, and voice box (larynx). In order to produce clear, "normal" speech, many quick, precise, coordinated movements take place. Producing speech involves four major components: 1) breathing (respiration), 2) making a sound/voicing (phonation), 3) forming speech sounds by using muscles like the lips and tongue (articulation), and finally, 4) adding rhythm and stress (prosody). When all of these components move and act smoothly, the result is clear, precise speech.

In dysarthria, any combination of the four components mentioned above can be affected, which can impact the following: 1) the quality and clarity of speech (e.g., speech can sound slurred, wet, breathy, or strained); 2) the pitch (e.g., whether your voice sounds low or high); 3) the volume (e.g., too loud or too quiet); 4) the speed (e.g., may speak very slowly); or 5) the melody of the speech (e.g., too flat or monotonous).

Just as in all other areas, dysarthria can range in severity from very mild to profound. The severity usually influences what is called "intelligibility," which typically is measured by how many words can be understood. In more severe cases, the person with dysarthria may speak so quietly that he or she cannot be heard, or makes no sound at all. These people would have significantly decreased intelligibility. In the most severe cases, the person with dysarthria may have difficulties being understood; their speech is "unintelligible." The good news is that asking the person with dysarthria to change something in their speech production usually results in improved intelligibility.

Evaluation

The SLP does an evaluation to decide if a person has dysarthria. There are many different types of dysarthria, depending on which of the four components discussed previously are impacted. The SLP determines what type of dysarthria the person has and then decides on an appropriate treatment plan. As always, the caregivers will play a crucial role in this process.

Treatment

Treatment for dysarthria is based on the results of the evaluation and information from the person with dysarthria and his or her caregivers. Treatment usually involves teaching the person with dysarthria and the caregivers some compensatory strategies to help improve not only speech intelligibility but also "comprehensibility," or the ability of others to comprehend the dysarthric individual. This approach requires looking not only at the speech of the person with dysarthria, but also at the whole picture, including the role of the communication partner and the environment. The SLP might suggest the following comprehensibility strategies:

For the Communication Partner of the Person with Dysarthria

- Make sure you know the general topic of conversation and use context to help increase understanding
- Choose the best time and place for communicating (e.g., not when the person is tired or distracted)
- Watch the speaker
- Eliminate/decrease environmental noise (e.g., turn off the TV, shut the door, etc.)
- Tune your ears; ask yes/no questions or give choices so you know what to listen for
- Ask the person with dysarthria to "get big" or "talk louder"
- Be specific about what you do not understand (e.g., "say that slower," "say that louder," "say that last part again," etc., is more specific than just "repeat that"). This approach will help the person with dysarthria conserve energy and make your communication more efficient.

For the Person with Dysarthria

- Get the listener's attention before you start talking
- Look straight at the listener when you talk

- Give the listener a general idea/context about what you're planning to say (e.g., "I want to talk about what I want for dinner.")
- Use gestures when appropriate
- Make sure the listener is following you; do not let them get lost
- Use a "backup system" in case of difficulty (e.g., paper and pencil or letterboard)

When dysarthria is more severe, people may need another way to communicate when he or she is not being understood. Some backup systems could include a piece of paper and a pencil to write key words, an alphabet board (to spell the word by pointing to the letters of the alphabet), or an electronic "talker". The SLP can help the person with dysarthria and their caregivers decide on an appropriate backup system.

KEY POINTS

- Speech therapy can help persons with brain injury learn to compensate for difficulties with thinking (cognition).
- Swallowing problems often occur after TBI. The SLP will help assess this problem and provide therapy to improve function. It is very important to follow the guidance of the SLP; otherwise, there is a risk of aspiration pneumonia.
- Neuropsychologists assess cognition through detailed testing and interview and provide strategies for recovery.

7

BEHAVIORAL AND EMOTIONAL EFFECTS OF BRAIN INJURY

TRESA ROEBUCK-SPENCER

[Ryan's] first word opened a floodgate of words. Ryan was complete-
ly uninhibited and verbalized whatever he was feeling. He cursed like
a sailor. I had never heard Ryan use foul language before and for the
next 72 hours his vocabulary was filled with expletives...Fortunately
for us, this behavior was short-lived, lasting all of 72 hours and never
rearing its ugly head again.   —Lorrie Knight-Major

As described in earlier chapters, a
brain injury can affect functioning in many areas. In the early stages of
recovery, many people pay the most attention to physical changes, such
as being able to use arms and legs and get around from place to place.
Over time, many people with brain injury regain physical abilities or
learn to do physical things in new ways. During this time, the individual
with a brain injury may behave and respond to things differently than he
or she did before. Sometimes a person with a brain injury may not even
realize that he or she is acting differently. Since each person and each
injury are different, not all people with injury will behave in the same
way. It is also important to remember that the way a person with brain
injury behaves while in the hospital may change as he or she recovers
and may change even more when he or she goes home from the hospital. Changes in behavior can present problems and can be upsetting to
family members and friends. Sometimes problem behaviors get better,
and sometimes they get worse. This section describes some of the most
common changes in behavior and emotions that can occur after brain

injury. Keep in mind that a given individual may not have any or all of these problems. The patient might also have problems that are not on this list. If you notice an unusual behavior change not listed here, be sure to ask the doctor, therapist, or psychologist.

AGITATION

Often early in the course of recovery, patients may become easily upset, difficult to console, and restless. During this state, patients may have trouble paying attention to what you are saying, and he or she may say or do things that do not make sense. Little things might get the patient angry, and it may be hard for him or her to calm down. He or she may have trouble sitting still and want to pace around the room or the unit. This condition is often referred to as agitation. Patients may have a tendency to become agitated when overstimulated (exposed to too much information at once) or tired. Sometimes painful procedures or confusing situations might lead to agitation. Agitation is common following brain injury, especially in the early stages of recovery. It is important to remember that this behavior can be a normal part of the recovery process. It often signals that the patient is improving from an unconscious or confused state to a more alert state.

What to Do When Agitation Is Observed

To avoid confusion when working with the patient, explain in simple statements who you are, what you are doing, how it will feel, and how long it will last. Keep the environment around the patient calm and quiet. Limit visitors to one or two at a time, and to individuals whom the patient knows well. Only one person should talk to the patient at a time. Do not try to talk to the patient at the same time that the nurse or therapist is talking to him. Do not talk on the phone or talk with other visitors while the doctor is talking with the patient. Keep the television or radio turned off, especially when visitors are present or the patient needs to pay attention to something. If it is noisy in the hallway, close the door. Keep visual stimulation to a minimum. One way to do this is to limit the number of pictures or cards that are hung on the walls. Although gifts are thoughtful, do not bring large colorful balloons or flower arrangements to the hospital because they can be distracting and overwhelming to the patient. Leave these gifts at home until the patient recovers to a point that these items are not overwhelming. If the patient becomes agitated or upset, talk to him or her in a calm, quiet voice and remove him or her from whatever is upsetting. Take the patient to a quiet place or ask others in the room to leave. These behaviors can be very upsetting, but it is very important not to argue with or yell at the patient.

DECREASED INITIATION: TROUBLE GETTING STARTED WITH THINGS

Often after a brain injury individuals may have trouble getting started with things. Therapists may refer to this as "decreased initiation," which happens because the pathways in the brain that help a person start a movement or task have been damaged. The patient may need extra help from others when beginning a task or help to keep going in the middle of a task after he or she has already started. In the hospital, a patient with this type of problem may have trouble starting a task when asked to and may just sit there without moving. For instance, if asked to put on his or her shoes, the patient may sit at the edge of the bed looking at the shoes without doing anything else. When asked to sign a piece of paper he or she may hold the pen and stare at the paper until prompted to sign. The patient may need reminders for each step of a multiple step task, such as brushing his or her teeth. Decreased initiation may look similar after discharge from the hospital. The person with decreased initiation may:

- Sit all day staring at the TV unless someone prompts him or her to do something else.
- Not seem interested in the things that the patient liked to do before.
- Not think to eat, bathe, brush his or her teeth, or perform other basic activities unless reminded.
- Not think of ideas for social activities or, if the patient has ideas, may not get started with them until reminded by someone else.
- Know what to do but just doesn't seem to be able to get started.

What to Do If Decreased Initiation Is Observed

Sometimes family members and friends may confuse decreased initiation with laziness or think that the patient with brain injury is not paying attention or trying hard enough. It is important to understand that decreased initiation is a common effect of brain injury and does not mean that the injured person is lazy. You can help the patient with brain injury by working with him or her to come up with a list of the steps needed to complete a task. You may need to help with this list, especially with the first few items. You can also make a checklist of the steps for routine activities to help the patient initiate and plan. It is important to remain calm. This behavior can get better with time. Sometimes medications can be helpful. Be sure to talk with the patient's doctor and psychologist if this behavior does not get better to see what other treatment options there might be.

LACK OF AWARENESS

In many cases a person with brain injury does not know that he or she is having problems. Or, the patient may realize that he or she has problems but thinks these problems are not a big deal. It is not unusual for a person with brain injury to appear to be in denial or ignoring the problems he or she is having. Someone with poor awareness may:

- Not seem concerned about his or her injury or the future, as if nothing is different.
- Insist that he or she can do things just as well as before the injury.
- Want to do activities that you know he or she cannot do.
- Complain that doctors, family members, and friends "don't know what they are talking about."
- Blame other people for the things that he or she cannot do. (For example, "I can go back to work, but the doctor won't let me.")
- Put himself or herself in dangerous situations because he or she does not understand his or her limitations.
- Not follow the recommendations made by the treatment team.

What to Do When Poor Awareness Is Observed

When a person has poor awareness it can be frustrating, but try to remain patient. Do not argue with a patient but instead calmly point out problems when they occur. Never yell or get angry. When it is safe, let the patient make mistakes on his or her own. This may sometimes be the only way to help him or her realize what problems are present. Talk things over with the patient after the mistake, and help him or her to think of ways to get around the problem the next time. Work with the patient to make good decisions and help him or her understand that, although he or she cannot do things he or she wants to right away (e.g., driving or staying home alone), he or she may be able to do some of these things after recovery. Help the patient to find alternative ways to do things (e.g., get a ride from friends) to decrease any frustration he or she may feel.

IMPULSIVITY: ACTING QUICKLY WITHOUT THINKING

Impulsivity describes when a person acts quickly, without thinking, about what he or she is doing or without thinking about the consequences of his or her actions. Impulsivity is a very common behavioral change after brain injury. It is usually worse in early stages of recovery and gets better over time. Impulsivity may remain in milder forms for a long time after injury and, for some, may be a persistent problem. Individuals with this problem may:

- Say whatever comes to mind without thinking first, even if it is offensive or rude to others.
- Do things without thinking of the consequences (for example, may attempt to return to work before he or she is ready).
- Do things that are dangerous or may lead to problems (for example, walking into the street without looking both ways, or spending all of his or her money on something he or she does not need).

What to Do When Impulsivity Is Observed

When you notice a person with brain injury acting without thinking, you can help by taking him or her aside and talking calmly about the consequences of what he or she is doing. You can also develop a signal that you use to let the patient know when he or she is doing something inappropriate in public. You can also help to plan ahead for social situations so that he or she does not overspend his or her budget.

LABILITY: OVERLY EMOTIONAL

Sometimes a person with a brain injury may react to situations with extreme emotions. The patient may appear to be laughing one minute and crying the next. He or she may laugh or cry more easily. He or she may laugh inappropriately when situations are not funny. For example, the patient may laugh when someone dies or is hurt, or when he or she is having trouble performing a task. He or she may cry over things that would not have been upsetting before.

What to Do When Emotional Lability Is Observed

When emotional lability happens, it can be confusing to the individual and those around him or her. Even though these reactions might be embarrassing, the patient is not doing it on purpose. So, it is important not to get upset. These extreme reactions can be part of the brain injury and are not the patient's fault. When emotional outbursts happen, try not to pay too much attention to this kind of behavior. Paying attention to such outbursts may increase the behavior. If possible, remove the thing that the patient is reacting to or remove him or her from the situation that triggered the emotion. Individuals with brain injury are often distracted easily so changing the topic of the conversation, or changing the television station, for example, can help to end the behavior. It is important to note that this problem may be worse in times of stress. Help the patient avoid stressful situations by working with him or her to plan ahead.

DEPRESSION

It is normal to sometimes feel sad or "down" after a brain injury.

Feelings of sadness are normal in stressful or difficult life situations. Generally, feelings of sadness come and go but do not significantly interfere with a person's motivation to do things or with his or her interest in seeing friends and family. Sometimes, feelings of sadness can worsen, and the patient may become depressed. Signs of depression include:

- Being sad a lot of the time and not being able to shake the feeling.
- Loss of interest in talking with or seeing other people.
- Loss of interest in things that were previously enjoyed.
- Difficulty falling or staying asleep OR sleeping too much. (Keep in mind that fatigue can also be a symptom of brain injury.)
- Decreased energy or motivation to do things. (Keep in mind that decreased initiation can also be a symptom of brain injury.)
- Decreased (or sometimes increased) appetite.
- Having recurrent thoughts of death or saying things like, "It would have been better if I had died in the accident . . .".

What to Do If Depression Is Observed

If there are concerns that the patient is depressed or becoming depressed, offer to talk with him or her about his or her feelings. Let the patient know that you support him or her and realize how much the injury has changed his or her life. If the person is still a patient in the hospital, talk with the doctor or psychologist about these signs of depression. There may be treatments (medicines, psychotherapy) that can help. If the person with injury is out of the hospital, it can help for him or her to get involved in activities that will take his or her mind off feeling sad. Social activities and exercise can be especially good. Activities that involve helping others may be especially helpful, but any increased activity would be good. If the injured person has many of the above signs of depression or talks about hurting himself or herself, you should contact his or her doctor or psychologist as soon as possible.

ANGER OR TEMPER OUTBURSTS

Following a brain injury, individuals often have trouble controlling their emotions. They may become angry or frustrated more easily than before or become angry in response to what others might think are small matters. Once angry, an individual with brain injury may have a more difficult time controlling what he or she says and does. This anger may become significant enough to lead to yelling, temper outbursts, and at times even physical actions or violence. One may have a difficult time preventing this; and once angry he or she may have trouble calming himself or herself down. Individuals with this problem may:

- Become angry easily over things that would not have upset him or her before.
- Raise his or her voice or yell a lot.
- Use bad language.
- Throw objects, hit things, or slam doors, etc.
- Hit, push, or otherwise hurt themselves or others.

What to Do If Anger Control Problems Are Observed

Prevention of anger outbursts is much easier then trying to calm down an individual after an outbreak occurs. Thus, prevention and watching for warning signs is the first line of defense. First, it is important to understand that being irritable and getting angry easily can be a result of brain injury. Try not to take these behaviors personally. Often patients become angry easily when they are agitated during the early stages of recovery. At this stage, the most important thing is to try to avoid situations that might upset the patient. Keep stimulation down. For example, keep the TV turned off. Stay calm. Do not argue with the patient. Limit the number of visitors at one time and the length of time that they visit. When possible, ignore bad behaviors like yelling or cursing. If needed, remove the patient from the situation. Paying too much attention to a behavior can sometimes make it worse. At later stages of recovery, it may be helpful to set up communication rules. Help the patient know that it is not acceptable to yell at, threaten, or hurt others when angry. Develop a signal that lets the patient know when his or her behavior is becoming out of control. Help the patient to recognize signs that he or she is becoming angry and to develop strategies for dealing with the anger, such as taking a deep breath and walking away. Talking with the patient's doctor or psychologist can also help when these behaviors seem like they are out of control.

INAPPROPRIATE OR EMBARRASSING BEHAVIOR

As mentioned above, it is often hard for individuals with a brain injury to control their emotions. It is also true that these individuals may have trouble controlling their behaviors, especially social behaviors, which can be very complex. This kind of behavior often leads to the patient's saying or doing things that are socially inappropriate and embarrassing. This behavior is usually caused by damage to parts of the brain that help us behave appropriately in social situations and help us to know when it is, and is not, appropriate to do and say things. For instance, most of us know when it is all right to make jokes and when it is not. We might say things among friends and family that we would not discuss at work or in more formal situations. Often, a person with brain injury may not be able to make these distinctions any longer and may treat all people and situations as familiar, even when he or she should behave in a more formal manner. Sometimes this behavior may be referred to as "disinhibition." Some examples of this type of behavior include:

- Telling strangers about personal matters that people are usually quiet about.
- Talking too long and not picking up on social cues that others are not interested.
- Asking personal questions of others he or she does not know well.
- Making inappropriate sexual comments or gestures in public.
- Using bad language excessively or at inappropriate times.

What to Do When Socially Inappropriate Behavior Occurs

Often the person with brain injury may not be aware that what he or she is doing or saying is inappropriate. When these behaviors occur, it is important to remain calm and not take it personally. These behaviors are often the result of the brain injury; the patient is not doing them on purpose. In a calm way, let him or her know that this behavior is wrong and that it bothers other people. Try not to pay too much attention to these behaviors. Paying too much attention or over-reacting to the problem can make it worse. Later in the recovery course or after the patient returns home, it may be helpful to come up with a signal to let the patient know when he or she is acting inappropriately. For example, you could hold up your hand to signal "stop," shake your head, "no," or say a special word that you have both agreed upon. Make sure you practice the signal ahead of time so that the patient knows what the signal means. Remember that the injury can make it hard for some individuals to act appropriately all the time, so it may not be realistic to expect the patient to have no inappropriate behaviors at all. For instance, he or she may be able to control some behaviors but not others, or he or she may be able to control his or her behavior in some situations but not in others. Remember that social interactions are very complex and take a lifetime to learn. When problems are present, you should work on one behavior at a time. Be sure to compliment the patient when he or she is successful in behaving appropriately. If inappropriate behaviors during a public outing are excessive or extreme, you may need to end the outing. If that happens, explain to the patient in a calm voice that you will have to end the outing because of a specific behavior. This explanation will help him or her to learn how to act appropriately when participating in social events with others.

KEY POINTS

- Emotional and behavioral changes are common after brain injury and may become more distressing to families and friends once the patient goes home from the hospital.
- Common problems include trouble getting started with things, lack of awareness, impulsivity, being overly emotional, depression, anger outbursts, and inappropriate or embarrassing behaviors.
- Not all patients show the same set of problem behaviors, and these behaviors may change over time as the patient recovers.
- When dealing with these behaviors, always remain calm and remember that the patient is not doing them on purpose. Overreacting can sometimes make the behavior worse.
- If you need help or have questions, talk to members of the patient's treatment team for recommendations.

8

CREATING A SAFE ENVIRONMENT

RHODA ONYIMA
CYNTHIA PINEDA

With their very practical support, my community helped deliver my
family from the abyss and ushered me into the next stage of recovery—
the post-hospital period.   —Rabbi Lynne Landsberg

Safety is a common area of concern
for caregivers and families following a brain injury. As you have experienced, observed or read in this book, brain injury can affect how a person moves, thinks, feels, and behaves depending on the area of the brain involved. Some of these changes may be temporary although some may persist depending on how the brain recovers. It is important during this period of recovery, that a safe environment is provided to the person who has sustained the brain injury as well as the people who are involved with his or her care. The purpose of this chapter is to provide the person with brain injury, and his or her caregivers, with basic information on the following:

- Causes and risks for falls following a brain injury.
- Tips on how to adjust the home environment to prevent falls.
- Use of restraints during hospitalization.
- Lifelong considerations for safety prevention.

Falls are a potentially catastrophic event, particularly in persons who have already sustained a brain injury. Severe consequences could result, such as another brain injury, fractures, fear of falling, and death. A number of factors lead to increased risk of falling following brain injury.

These can be grouped into two categories: factors that pertain to a person's physiological condition (intrinsic) and factors that address the physical environment (extrinsic). Examples of these risk factors are listed in Table 8.1.

Table 8.1 Risk factors for falls after a brain injury.

INTRINSIC Related to the Person's Condition	EXTRINSIC Related to the Environment

• Age (over 65 years old)
• Cognition (ability to think)
• Behavioral (impulsivity, agitation)
• Mobility, balance, and strength problems
• Visual and hearing difficulties
• Dizziness, lightheadedness
• Postural hypotension (low blood pressure when standing up)
• Incontinence
    - Bladder-inability to control urination
    - Bowel-inability to control stools
• Osteoporosis (weak bones)
• Anemia (low hemoglobin)
• Infections (such as in the urinary tract/bladder)
• Hypoglycemia (low glucose levels)
• Seizures
• Cardiac arrhythmias (slow or fast heart rates or irregular rhythms)
• Medications (sedatives)
	• Poor lighting
	• Wet or slippery floors
	• Throw rugs
	• Inadequate handrail support
	• Loose cords or wires
	• Inappropriate or lack of footwear
	• Low toilet seats
	• Broken equipment
	• Beds that are too high
	• Improper use or fit of canes, walkers, and wheelchairs
	• Wheels on beds or chairs
	• Cluttered rooms, floors, and staircases

PREVENTING FALLS

Remember that falls can be prevented, but they can still happen even to the most careful people or under the best of care given by caregivers and providers. We cannot control some risk factors, such as age and history of previous falls. An older person who has suffered a brain injury can have preexisting age-related changes that could contribute to the risk of falls. Some of these changes include visual difficulties (reduced vision because of cataracts or poor vision at night), decreased hearing, slower reaction response, urinary frequency, unsteady gait with impaired foot clearance, or decreased balance. However, we can do something about other risk factors to reduce the chance of falls. Developing a plan to decrease falls must be individualized. Such a plan takes a combination of medical treatment, rehabilitation and environmental changes. Interventions may include the following:

- Medical assessment after a fall to identify and address risk factors and treat underlying medical conditions; reviewing medications to assess side effects, risks, and benefits, and minimize use; encourage use of prescribed eyeglasses and hearing aids.
- Rehabilitation with physical therapy, occupational therapy, and speech therapy as appropriate to address balance, gait, strength, endurance, cognition, language, awareness, and behavior; assessment for, and proper use of, appropriate assistive mobility devices (wheelchairs, walkers, canes) and bathroom equipment.
- Home safety evaluation to review safety risks and modification of the environment to make it easier for persons with a brain injury to move around safely.
- Education of caregivers, family members, and staff members who provide care regarding fall risk factors and prevention strategies.

The modification of the environment is critical for prevention of falls. A number of potential environmental hazards, both indoor and outdoor, can contribute to accidental falls. The key areas that require evaluation are floor surfaces, steps, curbs, lighting, and grab bars. A common place where falls occur at home is the last step of the staircase. These falls may be caused by visual and perceptual disturbances. Interventions include teaching individuals to count steps and installing handrails. Table 8.2 provides some tips that can be used to create a safe home environment after a brain injury.

Behavioral and cognitive changes that occur after a brain injury may include agitation, impulsivity, poor judgment, and awareness. When combined with possible muscle weakness or imbalance, these changes could increase the risk of falling. If a person with a brain injury has physical or visual impairments that make walking difficult, speaking to the patient as he or she walks can further increase the risk of falling by causing a distraction. Impulsivity can also be an issue, so caregivers may need to remind the person with a brain injury to take his or her time. If outdoors, the patient should be instructed to avoid risk-taking behaviors, such as climbing on ladders. He or she should also pay close attention to the environment's uneven terrain and slippery surfaces.

RESTRAINT USE

Restraints consist of anything that restricts freedom of movement, including physical restraints such as vests, soft wrist ties, or full-length bed rails. Another means of restraining patients is with medications, usually sedatives, given to manage behavior. Medications that control behavior or cause sedation are not necessarily a restraint if used in an appropriate manner and in accordance with standard medical practice. Using restraints on a routine basis has not been shown to lower the risk of falls and injuries. Use of physical restraints could also lead to muscle weakness and deconditioning, which could further increase the risk of falling and injury. Restraints should only be used to provide safety during a period of imminent risk of self-injury or injury to others during the recovery period of the person with a brain injury. The person's rights, dignity, and well-being will be respected and considered when the use of a restraint is determined to be a necessary component of the treatment plan. A restraint must not be used for the purposes of coercion, discipline, convenience, or retaliation. The following guidelines are usually followed by hospitals:

- Restraints will only be used when alternative techniques have failed or have been considered and deemed inappropriate.
- The least restrictive restraint will be used.

Table 8.2 Modifications to create a safe home environment:

Area of Home/Environment	Modifications
Lighting	Install glow-in-the-dark light switches at the top and bottom of stairways and place a night-light along the route between the bedroom and bathroom. Keep a flashlight and new batteries by the bed in case of a power outage.
Flooring and Footwear	Keep appliance, lamp, and telephone cords out of areas where you walk. Do not put cords under rugs. Wear proper footwear at all times, even inside the home. Never walk around with just socks or stockings on your feet. Avoid high heels or platform shoes.
Bathroom	Use a rubber mat or put adhesive texture strips on the bottom of the tub or shower. Install grab bars on the walls for additional support. Place a slip-resistant rug on tile floors to safely get in and out of the bathtub. Avoid bar soaps. Use liquid soap from a dispenser mounted in the shower.
Stairways/Steps	Install rails on both sides of staircases if possible. Adhere nonslip threads to bare wood steps, and remove small area rugs at the top and bottom of the stairs. Paint the last step a different color, indoors and outdoors.
Kitchen	Use a step stool or reacher, not chairs or boxes, to reach items in upper cabinets. Clean up kitchen spills immediately. Use nonskid kitchen floor wax.
Bedroom	Stabilize beds and bedside furniture. Clear pathways between bedroom and bathroom. Keep objects within reach to avoid overreaching.

- Use of restraints is based on the individual person's needs and limited to clinically justified situations.
- Only staff determined to be competent will apply restraints.
- Monitoring and reassessment are done by staff trained in restraint use.
- Physical and emotional needs will be met during restraint use.
- Brain-injured individuals and their families will be involved in the plan to use, reduce, and eliminate restraints.

The decision to use a restraint is based on clinical observation by the physician and the other members of the rehabilitation team. Persons for whom restraints are being used should be checked frequently to ensure safety and proper application of the restraint and to make sure that the call system and bed position control devices are within reach. Caregivers should ensure that the person in restraints has access to adequate fluid and is offered assistance with toileting or any other care needs every 2 hours while awake. In a hospital, care issues addressed during a period of restraint use may include taking vital signs, performing range of motion exercises, repositioning, checking circulation, and checking skin for any evidence of breakdown. The need for continued use of restraints is reassessed daily by members of the rehabilitation team.

What Are Alternatives to the Use of Restraints?

When behaviors cannot be modified, some alternatives to restraints are used in a rehabilitation setting. Some persons with a brain injury who are confused or agitated may try to remove intravenous (IV) lines, feeding tubes, trach (tracheostomy) tubes, etc. Sometimes covering an IV site with a bandage or using an abdominal binder to cover the feeding tube will be effective and eliminate the need for restraints. People who become more agitated by restraints, or who are able to get themselves out of restraints, may benefit from one-to-one supervision. Family members can assist with this effort.

A person with a brain injury who is physically safe to walk around may benefit from this activity and it may also help reduce agitation. However, the person who is confused and wanders into other people's rooms or tries to leave the unit may require restraints. If, however, it is safe for a person to walk independently, it is preferable to encourage walking rather than using restraints. Nursing call bells should be placed within reach of the patient. Other devices, such as bed alarms, may also reduce the need for restraints. Both in the hospital and at home, keeping a person who is at risk of falling in view of others can help prevent falls, reduce agitation, and potentially avoid the need for restraints.

QUIET SPACES

Overstimulation is frequently a trigger for agitation and aggression. It is important to minimize stimulating the person with a brain injury. There are several ways to avoid overstimulation. When the person is still an inpatient at the hospital, visitors should be limited to just two or three at a time, and they should avoid all speaking at once. Keep conversations to one at a time. If there is a conversation going on, turn off the television or radio and keep other distractions to a minimum. If there is a roommate who also has visitors, it may be easier to go to a quiet location where the brain injury survivor and his or her visitors can talk. If there is much noise or visual stimulation occurring, it may be necessary for caregivers or staff members to escort the person to a quiet room where he or she can sit and watch TV, talk to someone, or just rest to avoid a behavioral problem. It is a good idea to have a quiet space at home, too. Many family members or friends at the house may be too stimulating, so the patient may need somewhere to relax without being disturbed.

In public places, such as shopping malls and restaurants, it may be more difficult to find a quiet space. Therefore, caregivers should look for potential areas that may be suitable for a rest break for the person with a brain injury to escape the stimulating environment.

ASSISTIVE DEVICES

Walking aids, such as canes, walkers, and crutches may be helpful devices that can help with one's mobility after a brain injury. It is important to remember not to use or borrow someone else's device as they may not be the right type or size. Friends and family members, who have an old walking aid they are no longer using, will often give them to the person with a brain injury. The device should still be evaluated by a therapist before use to ensure proper size and type. Also, the person should know how to properly use it. If the patient does use a cane or walker prescribed for him or her, check that the rubber tips are not worn and that it is adjusted to his or her height. Falls from wheelchairs are also common. Use the seatbelt and apply the brakes when needed. Be cautious during transfers. The proper use and fit of wheelchairs will help prevent other injuries.

WHAT TO DO AFTER A FALL

As mentioned above, some falls will occur despite the best preventive measures. Here are some recommended techniques for the person who has fallen to follow after the fall:

- If possible, try to fall on your side or buttocks. Roll over naturally, turning your head in the direction of the roll.
- Keep your wrists, elbows, and knees bent. Do not try to break the fall with your hands or elbows.
- If you feel you are not injured and are able to get up, crawl to a strong and stable piece of furniture, like a chair, that you can use as a support to help pull yourself up. Put both hands on the seat and slowly begin to raise yourself up. Bend whichever knee is stronger, keeping the other knee on the floor. Finally, slowly twist and sit in the chair. Call a family member or friend to check and make sure there are no injuries.
- If you feel you have suffered an injury, do not try to get up. Take several deep breaths after falling. Call 911 or a family member for help.

The skin should be inspected for any breaks, discoloration, or swelling. Pain in any body part suggests possible injury to that area. Medical examination and x-rays may be indicated if a fracture or other serious injury is suspected. However, it is important to note that fractures or internal bleeding in the brain (if you hit your head) may not readily be apparent immediately after a fall. If a person who has fallen thinks that he or she has hit his or her head, someone should contact the physician immediately so that careful examination, observation and prompt treatment can be done if needed.

LIFELONG SAFETY CONSIDERATIONS

Other questions often arise surrounding safety in the following situations: resuming recreational sports, driving, sexual activity, living alone, working, and managing finances and medications. The other chapters in this book will help the person with a brain injury and his or her caregivers with these concerns. While it is important to focus on maximizing the person's capabilities at home and the community, lifelong prevention is key to avoid further injury to the brain and body as the person recovers from the initial brain injury. Examples include using seatbelts and helmets. The use of alcohol and drugs should be avoided as these substances can impair thinking and recovery. While creating a "brain injury friendly environment" may be a daunting task, remember that the brain injury survivor is not alone on the road to recovery. The rehabilitation team (i.e., doctors, psychologists, nurses, therapists, social worker, support groups, and caregivers) is there to assist and advocate for success in living well with your brain injury.

KEY POINTS

- A brain injury can affect how a person moves, thinks, feels and behaves.
- Cognitive and physical changes along with older age, physiological changes, and use of medications can contribute to the risk of falls and should be frequently assessed to minimize the risk of falls.
- Restraints should be used only when indicated and after alternative measures have been considered.
- Safety is everyone's responsibility and lifelong prevention is key to avoid further injury to oneself and others.

9

MEDICATIONS COMMONLY USED IN THE TREATMENT OF BRAIN INJURY

MICHAEL R. YOCHELSON

Tone is a bitch (before her Baclofen pump) . . . *I feel like a wet noodle* (after her Baclofen pump)   —Selina Brijbasi

When medications are discussed in this chapter and throughout the book, the trade (brand) name and generic names will be given together initially. Then the name used most frequently among hospital staff will be used so that the reader will be able to associate it with what he or she is being told by physicians and other staff.

A number of different medications are commonly used in the management of persons with brain injuries. Most of the medications are not specific to the type of brain injury. They may be used for most any acquired brain injury, to include traumatic brain injury, anoxic or hypoxic brain injury, subarachnoid hemorrhage from the rupture of an aneurysm or AVM, etc. The medications discussed in this chapter are grouped according to the primary symptoms which they treat in brain injury; however, several of the medications may have multiple uses. Additionally, the list is not exhaustive. Extensive research is being carried out in the field of brain injury, and new drugs are frequently being used in the management of people with brain injuries.

Note that all medications have the potential for side effects. As an inpatient, side effects are monitored, and medications and/or doses are adjusted accordingly. It is always advisable to be aware of the possible side effects and medication interactions of the drugs you take. Read the package inserts or discuss your medications with your pharmacist or physician. If it is believed that the person taking the medication is having an adverse side effect the physician should be notified immediately. If a serious allergic reaction occurs, such as rash, swelling, hives, difficulty breathing, the medication should be stopped immediately and emergency medical assistance should be sought. However, if the person has a more common side effect (*not* allergic reaction), it is advisable to discuss stopping the medication with the physician *before* stopping it because some medications have more serious consequences if stopped abruptly. It should also be noted that occasionally physicians use the side effects of a medication to benefit the patient.

AGITATION AND BEHAVIORAL PROBLEMS

Probably the most common group of medications used to help reduce agitation and irritability include antipsychotics. Many people are reluctant to take antipsychotics, or their families are hesitant to allow them to be given to the brain-injured person because they are afraid of their "mind-altering properties" and/or the social stigma associated with them. However, antipsychotic medications are often a very important part of the recovery and management of people with brain injuries. When prescribed and taken properly, they can be very effective. These medications help to control abnormal thought processes, such as hallucinations, delusions, and paranoia, which can occur after a brain injury. They also help to reduce agitation and calm the person after a brain injury. Most people need to take these only for a short period of time, days to weeks; but occasionally they may need to take them for months, years, or even permanently.

Antipsychotics can be divided into two groups. The older (or first generation) antipsychotics, such as Haldol™ (haldoperidol), tend to have more side effects, in particular abnormal movements (so-called "extrapyramidal side effects"). These side effects can be decreased somewhat by also administering an antihistamine such as Cogentin™ (benztropine) or Benadryl (diphenhydramine) with the antipsychotic. Newer antipsychotics tend to have fewer side effects. These include such medications as Seroquel™ (quetiapine), Zyprexa™ (olanzepine), Risperdal™ (risperidone), Abilify™ (aripiprazole), and Geodon™

(ziprasidone). In addition to helping with agitation, these medications are sometimes used to help with sleep, particularly if the person with the brain injury has confusion and restlessness in the evenings ("sun downing").

Depending on the particular medication, side effects can be quite variable. Some of the more common ones include headaches, fatigue, changes in blood pressure or heart rate, light headedness, weight gain, and elevated liver enzyme levels.

DEPRESSION AND MOOD DISORDERS

Antidepressants are the primary group of medications used to help control depression. However, there are other groups of medications that can help with mood as well. Several classes of antidepressants are used in the management of a depressed person with a brain injury. The first choice would be a selective serotonin reuptake inhibitor, or "SSRI." The one in this group that has been most studied and shown to be not only helpful with depression, but also with motor and cognitive processing speed in people with brain injuries is Zoloft™ (sertraline). Zoloft™ is considered somewhat activating, so it is also helpful for people who have mild fatigue or decreased initiation or motivation following a brain injury. Some other SSRIs that may be used include Prozac™ (fluoxetine), Paxil™ (paroxetine), Celexa™ (citalopram), and Lexapro™ (escitalopram). The main side effects noted with these medications include gastrointestinal (GI) symptoms, such as nausea or diarrhea, and sexual dysfunction including decreased libido. Many of the side effects are dose-related (occur more frequently or more intensely with increasing doses) and/or self-limited (resolve with time). Therefore, unless the person taking the medication is having a serious reaction, it would be best to try to continue the medication to see if it becomes more tolerable.

While SSRIs are the most commonly used antidepressants among people with brain injuries, there are other types of antidepressants. Serotonin noradrenergic reuptake inhibitors ("SNRIs") include Effexor™ (venlafaxine) and Cymbalta™ (duloxetine). These medications are effective in the management of depression in this population. In addition, they have an added benefit of reducing neuropathic pain. They have primarily been studied in pain resulting from abnormalities in the peripheral nervous system (e.g., painful diabetic neuropathy);

however, it is our experience that they also help with central neuropathic pain (pain resulting from injury to the central nervous system).

Tricyclic antidepressants, such as Elavil™ (amitriptyline), Pamelor™ (nortryptiline), and others are rarely used as primary antidepressants in the brain injury population. They have a tendency to cause excessive sedation and slow cognitive skills. However, occasionally they are used at low doses to help with reducing headache frequency or neuropathic pain. (See section on headache medications below.) Another reason that these antidepressants are often avoided in this population of patients is that tricyclic antidepressants ("TCAs") lower seizure threshold. People who have suffered a brain injury are already at increased risk for seizures.

Wellbutrin™ (bupropion) is another antidepressant which is occasionally used. It is an effective antidepressant and docs not have the sexual side effects of the SSRIs; in fact, sometimes if taken in conjunction with SSRIs, it can reduce the SSRI's effect on the libido. However, like TCAs, Wellbutrin™ can lower the seizure threshold so it must be used with caution. In addition to the antidepressants, some antiepileptic drugs ("AEDs," anticonvulsants, seizure medications) can help with mood stabilization. These are particularly useful in patients who may have a prior history of mania or bipolar disorder (manic depression) because the SSRIs can occasionally cause a person to go from a depressed state to mania with significant agitation, particularly among people with brain injuries. The most common seizure medications used to address controlling mood include Depakote™ (divalproic acid, valproic acid) and Lamictal™ (lamotrigine).

ANXIETY

Anxiolytics are medications used to control anxiety. Anxiety is a common problem after brain injury. Furthermore, patients who have underlying anxiety disorders may have their anxiety symptoms made worse by the brain injury. Some of the SSRI antidepressants, such as Zoloft™, also have properties that help control anxiety and are often the first line of treatment for anxiety because they also help with mood. Benzodiazepines, such as Valium™ and Ativan™, are commonly used to treat anxiety. These medications are usually avoided in patients with severe cognitive impairment as they are CNS depressants and can cause mental status changes. However, these medications do have the benefit of being available in injectable (intravenous/IV and intramuscular/IM) forms so they can be given to a patient who cannot take oral medications and/or someone who is very agitated and unwilling to take medications. The benzodiazepines also can act as muscle relaxants, which can be beneficial in patients with spasticity. BuSpar™ (buspirone) is a pure anxiolytic that is generally well tolerated and can be used in patients with significant anxiety, but without the need to treat depression. Lyrica™ (pregabalin) has been shown to be effective in patients with anxiety and should be considered in patients with seizures or nerve pain.

ATTENTION, AROUSAL AND FATIGUE

Medications for arousal (alertness) are an important part of the early rehabilitation in people who are at a very low level as a result of brain injury. One group of medications commonly used affect dopamine receptors. Dopamine is a chemical in the brain that affects arousal. These medications include Parlodel™ (bromocriptine), Sinemet™ (carbidopa/levodopa), and Symmetrel™ (amantadine). More recently, some physicians are using Azilect™ for arousal. Some limited studies would suggest that Ambien™, a medicine used to help sleep, actually improves arousal in lower level brain injury patients.

Attention is distinct from arousal in that it is the ability of a person to focus on a subject for a period of time. Neurostimulants are helpful in improving attention. Some of these include Ritalin™ (short acting methylphenidate), Concerta™ or Metadate™ (long-acting methylphenidate), Dexedrine™ (dextroamphetamine), Strattera™ (atomoxetine), and Adderall™ (amphetamine/dextroamphetamine). These medications are generally well tolerated but can cause changes in blood pressure and heart rate; they can also make some people feel jittery.

These stimulants are also useful in treating fatigue, which is a very common problem in TBI, even after mild TBI. In addition, Provigil™ (modafinil) is frequently prescribed. Provigil™ has fewer cardiac side effects. Although Provigil™ does not change the long-term outcome after brain injury, it can help the recovery in the acute period because the person who had a brain injury is less tired and better able to tolerate intensive therapy.

HEADACHES

Headaches are one of the most common symptoms following every severity level of traumatic brain injury. Many people will just have post-traumatic headaches for a short period of time (days to a few weeks), but others may suffer with this problem for months, years, or indefinitely. Two general categories of medications are used in the treatment of headaches: (1) prophylactic medications taken daily to reduce the severity and frequency of headaches; and (2) abortive medications used on an as-needed basis to control a headache.

The medications used for prophylactic treatment include certain anticonvulsants (seizure medications), antidepressants, and blood pressure medications. In the TBI population, anticonvulsants may be the best choice since the other groups may have more unwanted side effects. The antidepressants used (tricyclic antidepressants) are very sedating. They also have other side effects that should be considered before using these medications. The blood pressure medications may be well tolerated, especially in people with mild brain injury. But for those with more severe injury, they may already have very low, or difficult to control, blood pressure that may be an issue if using these drugs. The advantage of using anticonvulsants is that they provide protection against seizures and help reduce headaches. A number of the anticonvulsants also have mood stabilization properties that may be beneficial as well.

The first line for post-traumatic headache abortive should be an NSAID (non-steroidal anti-inflammatory drug), such as Motrin™ (ibuprofen) or Tylenol™ (acetaminophen), early in the course until it is established how frequently headaches occur or if they respond to these milder medications. In the early post-trauma period, narcotics can be used for more severe pain. However, these should be used only for a limited period of time. If the need persists, doctors should consider adding prophylactic medications and changing to a non-narcotic pain medicine.

PAIN MEDICATIONS

This section will discuss management of non-headache pain. Pain following a traumatic brain injury can generally be divided into neuropathic (nerve) pain and nociceptive (bone, muscle, and soft tissue) pain. One of the more common underlying causes of persistent pain is spasticity. The first line of treatment for this problem is management of the spasticity which should, in turn, reduce the pain. In conjunction with anti-spasticity medications, NSAIDs, Tylenol™, or narcotics may be prescribed.

For nociceptive pain, one should always try to use the mildest, non-addictive, pain medications. If narcotics are necessary for a prolonged period, long-acting scheduled (not "as needed") medications should be considered. However, for people who have a feeding tube, the long-acting medications may not be an option since they cannot be crushed. The fentanyl patch is a long-acting narcotic that would be an option. The patch is applied to the skin every 3 days and provides a slow, continuous dose of medicine. Ultram™ is another medication that works at the same receptor as narcotics, but is milder. However, it can lower the seizure threshold and, therefore, should be used with caution in persons with brain injury.

For neuropathic pain, there are many helpful medications. Some of these include Cymbalta™, Lyrica™, Neurontin™ (gabapentin), and tricyclic antidepressants. The specific medications used will depend upon many factors, to include cause of pain, associated symptoms, other medications the person is already taking, etc. It should be understood that all of these medications are also used for other diseases (e.g., depression, seizures). They are used to reduce pain by taking them on a daily basis; they usually will not be effective if used "as needed."

BOWEL AND BLADDER MANAGEMENT

After a severe brain injury, it is common to have some bowel problems, particularly constipation. This problem may be caused by the injury itself, causing a neurogenic bowel, or it can be a result of side effects from other medications (especially narcotics). A person with TBI who is having bowel problems should be on a regular regimen of stool softeners, fiber (bulking) agents, or laxatives. If the problem is severe enough, this regimen may include regular use of a suppository or enema. Many such medications are available, most over the counter. Some of the common medications used in controlling bowel function include Colace™ (docusate), Senna, Metamucil™, and Miralax™ (polyethylene glycol), which are taken by mouth. Dulcolax™ (bisacodyl) is available orally and by suppository. An enema is the introduction of liquid in the rectum. Some enemas are commercially available and are commonly used in a hospital and available over the counter, such as Fleet™ (sodium phosphate) enemas. An alternative to commercially available enemas is the use of a soapsuds enema, which is very effective.

A neurogenic bladder can also occur. This may be partially caused by prolonged use of a Foley catheter, which puts the bladder at rest; it can also be caused by the brain injury itself. General management is discussed in Chapter 5. Several different classes of medications are used to control a neurogenic bladder. The correct one depends on why the person has a neurogenic bladder. This is important to determine because the wrong type of medication could make the symptoms worse. The most important thing to watch for is urinary retention (inability to urinate). Some medications used include Bentyl™ (dicyclomine hydrochloride), Ditropan™ (oxybutinin), and Detrol™ (tolterodine).

SEIZURES

Seizures are discussed in more detail in Chapter 2. Here we will just discuss some of the medications used to treat seizures. Essentially any anticonvulsant may be helpful in the treatment of post-traumatic epilepsy. However, some medications are used more commonly because they have been studied in greater detail or they have fewer side effects in this population. For years, Dilantin™ (phenytoin) was the drug of choice for treating and preventing post-traumatic seizures. In part, this was the drug of choice because it is available in an intervenous (IV) formula so the doctor can give it to a person who is not able to take pills. Blood levels can be measured, which also helps the clinician to ensure that the patient is getting enough drug. However, Dilantin™ has many side effects, both short- and long-term, which limit its use. A drug rash from Dilantin™ is an allergic reaction and requires the medication to be discontinued immediately. Other side effects that are not as severe, but still have an impact on the rehabilitation of a person with a brain injury, include slowing down cognitive processing.

Similar to IV Dilantin™ is Cerebyx™ (phosphenytoin). This is a "pro-drug," which breaks down into Dilantin™ after it is in the body. However, it is easier to administer as it can be given at a faster rate since it does not hurt the blood vessels as much and does not cause hypotension. This medication is usually only used to "load" a patient or for a patient in status epilepticus.

Keppra™ (levitiracitam) is now one of the most commonly used anticonvulsants for post-traumatic seizure prevention. It is very useful because it can be started at a full-strength (therapeutic) dose, whereas other medications must be slowly titrated to a therapeutic dose to avoid side effects. Keppra™ has also recently become available as an IV medication, which is helpful for those people who require IV medications.

Among the older anticonvulsants, such as Dilantin™, are phenobarbital, Depakote™, and Tegretol™ (carbamazepine). Phenobarbital is rarely used in the adult population due to sedation. Depakote™ is frequently used because it has the advantage of mood stabilization, but it must be used with great caution in women of child-bearing age as it can cause birth defects. Tegretol™ is also sometimes used, especially if the person with brain injury is also having shooting pains from a nerve injury. Certain labs and blood levels of the medications must be monitored with each of the medicines mentioned above.

Since 1993, there have been many new anticonvulsants, to include Keppra™, on the market. In general, these medicines have fewer side effects and do not require the same degree of monitoring through blood tests. This group of medicines includes Trileptal™ (oxcarbazepine), which is similar to Tegretol™; therefore, if a person has side effects from Tegretol, caution should be used if trying Trileptal™. Lamictal™ is another medication that is being used more often in brain injury. Like Depakote™, it has the advantage of being a mood stabilizer. Extreme caution must be used if using Lamictal™ and Depakote™ together because of an increased risk of severe rash. If a rash does occur, the medication should be stopped immediately and the prescribing physician contacted. Lyrica™ has been used in this population as an adjunct (add-on) medication, but it has not been studied as monotherapy (single drug treatment) for post-traumatic seizures. However, it may be useful as an add-on medication for certain people because it can help to decrease certain types of nerve pain.

See Table 9.1 for a complete list of seizure medications. It should be noted that benzodiazepines, such as Ativan™ (lorazepam), are also effective anticonvulsants. They are usually used to stop a seizure, rather than as seizure prophylaxis. They are not listed in Table 9.1.

Table 9.1 Antiepileptic (anti-seizure) drugs.

Trade Name	Generic Name	Common Uses*
Depakote™ Depakene™** Divalproate™	divalproic acid valproic acid sodium valproate	Seizures Mood stabilization
Dilantin™**	phenytoin	Seizures Neuropathic pain
Felbatol™	felbamate	Seizures†
Gabatril™	tiagabine	Seizures Panic disorder
Keppra™**	levitiracitam	Seizures
Lamictal™	lamotrigine	Seizures Mood stabilization PTSD
Luminal™	phenobarbital	Seizures
Lyrica™	pregabalin	Seizures Neuropathic pain Fibromyalgia
Neurontin™	gabapentin	Neuropathic pain Seizures
Tegretal™ Carbatrol™	carbamazepine	Seizures Trigeminal neuralgia Mood stabilization Phantom limb pain
Topamax™	topiramate	Seizures Migraine Pseudotumor cerebri***

Table 9.1 (continued) Antiepileptic (anti-seizure) drugs.

Trileptal™	oxcarpazepine	Seizures Trigeminal neuralgia Mood stabilization
Vimpat™**	lacosamide	Seizures Tremor
Zonegran™	zonisamine	Seizures

* Not all uses listed are FDA approved.
** Available in IV form.
*** Weak carbonic anhydrase inhibitor;
    may be useful for pseudotumor cerebri.
† High risk medication; requires written consent before using;
    not recommended for post-traumatic epilepsy.

SLEEP

Sleep problems are a common issue after a brain injury. There are many options to help with sleep. The key to good sleep is determining why someone is not sleeping well and treating the underlying problem. In this section, the medications are those used most commonly for insomnia. However, sometimes, a person does not sleep well because of pain, anxiety, or some other issues. These other problems should be the focus of treatment.

Desyryl™ (trazodone) is one of the most commonly used medications to treat insomnia in the brain-injured person. It is an antidepressant, but it is the sedative effect that helps with the insomnia. Use of trazodone for sleep does not automatically imply that the patient has depression.

Since many medications have sedation as a side effect, it is often possible to give a medication at bedtime, which is being used to treat another issue, and have it successfully treat insomnia. If a person still has difficulty sleeping, some of the newer sleep aids can be used. These include Ambien™ or Ambien CR™ (zolpidem), Lunesta™ (eszopiclone), Sonata™ (zaleplon), or Rozerem™ (ramelteon). Although studies regarding treating insomnia in TBI are limited, this author prefers to add Rozerem™, which acts at the melatonin receptor in the body. Melatonin is a hormone that the human body makes; it is involved in controlling the sleep-wake cycle. Rozerem™, like melatonin, can help to maintain a normal circadian rhythm (sleep-wake cycle).

SPASTICITY

A common problem after more severe traumatic brain injury includes spasticity. Spasticity, or increased muscle tone, is discussed in the chapter on physical and occupational therapy (Chapter 5). In this chapter, we will discuss the medications that will help to reduce spasticity. Oral spasticity medications include Liorisal™ (baclofen), Zanaflex™ (tizanidine), and Dantrium™ (dantrolene). Others are used with variable effect, but these are the three most common drugs. The first two can cause significant drowsiness and central nervous system (CNS) depression. Dantrolene can also act this way, but to a lesser degree. Zanaflex™ can lower blood pressure, which can be beneficial for some people, but may be a problem if the blood pressure is already very low. In addition to the oral medications, botulinum toxin (e.g., Botox™ or Myobloc™) can be injected into selected muscles to reduce spasticity. This medication can be very helpful, but because of a maximum dose limitation, it is only helpful for focused treatment not for generalized spasticity. Intrathecal baclofen is another option. This option involves an implantable pump that delivers baclofen directly to the spine. The benefit of the pump is that it allows for more effective control of spasticity than oral baclofen without the sedating side effect. The disadvantage is that it requires a surgical procedure. It also requires seeing a specialized doctor/clinic for refills of the pump every one month to six months.

GENERAL MEDICAL CONDITIONS

Other general medical conditions, such as high blood pressure, heart rhythm changes, diabetes, and thyroid problems, should be managed with the same medications as one would use without a TBI. However, the prescribing doctor must be aware of drug-drug interactions with new drugs that one may be taking for the TBI and associated symptoms. The doctor should also be familiar with the side effects of the medications that could make the symptoms of the TBI worse, especially fatigue and cognitive impairment.

KEY POINTS

- No medications are specifically FDA approved for TBI. Therefore, understand that the doctors treating TBI often use medications for "off label" uses. That approach does not mean that they are unsafe.
- Often multiple medications can be used for the same problem; therefore, it is important to pay attention to side effects and drug interactions to determine the best treatment option for a given individual.

—10—
EFFECTS OF BRAIN INJURY ON FAMILY, SOCIAL ROLES, AND CAREGIVER ISSUES

TRESA ROEBUCK-SPENCER
JUDSON RICHARDSON

There is no question that this experience has changed our family. We are a kindler, gentler family now. Knowing that at any second everything in your life can change makes you more aware of each other, more respectful of feelings. —Sharon Douglas

A brain injury can affect the way the brain normally works. After an injury, the nerve cells in the brain may become damaged and unable to send information to each other the way they did in the past. Changes in the brain can result in changes to a person's behavior and abilities. Not all people experience the same problems after an injury. It may take a long time before a person with brain injury gets better and returns to previous activities. Some people may never be able to return to all of the activities they did before the injury, but they may be able to return to some. They might also be able to return to some activities, but they may have to do them in a different way.

Depending on the type and severity of brain injury, a person with brain injury may go through a series of changes over time with the most severe changes seen soon after the injury. These problems typically improve over time. Although most problems improve, it is not possible to predict how much improvement will occur or how long recovery will take.

Watching someone you care about recover from a brain injury can be very stressful and emotional. It might be possible to control your emotions when you are at the hospital, but when you are alone, you may begin to feel overwhelmed. The closer you are to the person with brain injury, the more overwhelmed you may feel. It may be comforting to know that these feelings are normal. Below is a list of some common feelings you might experience after someone you know has a brain injury:

- Shock. Feelings of shock include numbness, confusion, and fear. Many people also feel helpless. You may find yourself thinking, "I must be dreaming. This can't happening!"
- Denial. During denial, you may not be able to realize or admit what has happened and that life has changed. Denial is a normal way to cope with the reality of a devastating situation. You may find yourself thinking, "The doctors don't know what they are talking about. My loved one will be OK in a few weeks."
- Sadness or Despair. As you begin to accept what has happened, the reality may be overwhelming. You may feel that this is the worst thing that could happen and wonder how you will go on. You may think, "My life is over. Nothing will ever be the same." You should not feel guilty or ashamed of these feelings. They are normal reactions. These feelings help you to accept and face the situation. Most people have to experience these feelings before they can get through them.
- Blame. Another common reaction is to blame someone. You may feel sure that this was someone's fault. Some people even start blaming the doctor or other members of the healthcare team. Again, this can be a normal part of feeling sad about losing the person you knew before the brain injury and accepting the changes that you see now.
- Mobilization. It can be comforting to have a plan and feel like you have some control over the situation. You might find yourself saying, "I'm ready to learn. How can I help?"
- Grief. You may find yourself missing the old person and the times you spent together. Grieving is not only painful for family and caregivers but also for the injured person. Most people with brain injury want their old life back, too.
- Anger or Resentment. A person with brain injury needs to focus on getting better. He or she may not be able to do the things he or she

used to and may need your help to do things he or she was able to do well before his or her injury. The person with the injury may require your help to get better, and he or she will be less available to help you. You may end up with more responsibilities and more stress. This can lead to anger and resentment. These feelings are normal but can sometimes make you feel guilty. If you have these feelings, you may need to take a break and ask others for help.

- Guilt. Some people may have survivor's guilt and feel bad that the other person was hurt instead of them. They may say that they wish they could trade places with the injured person. Some people may feel guilt at not having prevented the injury and spend hours wondering what they should have done to prevent the injury (e.g., "I should never have let him drive."). Finally, some people might take blame for incomplete recovery and feel that the injured person would have gotten better if they could only do more for them. Because of guilt feelings, family members or friends may feel that they should focus 100% of their effort and time on the patient. Remember, though, that everyone needs rest, and that taking care of yourself is one of the most important things after the injury.

- Depression. Sadness and despair can be normal reactions when someone you know has had a brain injury. Sometimes these feelings may develop into depression. Depression can be serious, especially if you get so depressed that you do not feel like eating, have trouble sleeping and caring for yourself or your family. If you find yourself feeling this way, talk with someone and let them know how you are feeling. You can even talk with someone on the healthcare team and ask for help. It is important to deal with these feelings before they get out of control. If you start to have thoughts of death or hurting yourself, you should talk to someone, preferably a doctor or psychologist immediately.

- Anxiety or Worry. It is common to worry when a friend or family member has had a brain injury. You may find yourself thinking, "How will we ever pay for all these bills?" "What if they don't get better?" "How am I going to handle this?" Worry is normal. Signs of more significant worries or anxiety include trouble sleeping, feelings of restlessness, racing heart, irritability, and panic attacks. If you begin to notice significant anxiety, talk to someone on the healthcare team and ask for help.

Everyone handles stress in different ways. You might feel some of the emotions listed above, or even all of them, at one point or another. It is important to remember that these feelings are normal. Recommendations later in this chapter will help caregivers deal with these reactions when they occur.

WHAT SHOULD I EXPECT WHEN WE GO HOME?

Going home from the hospital can be exciting and scary at the same time. This may be a time when the patient and caregivers are relieved that the worst is over and that they are ready to get away from the hospital and back to familiar surroundings. It can also be a scary time. Some patients and caregivers may have developed bonds with the therapists, doctors, and nurses, and they may worry about leaving the structure of the hospital. It is normal to worry about how things will be different after discharge from the hospital. It is hard to know what to expect when the injured person goes home. The effects of brain injury are complicated and hard to understand. Often people who have had a brain injury act very differently than they did before. The physical changes are often the most obvious in the beginning. Changes in personality and emotional well-being may not be noticeable until later. Sometimes these problems are not realized until the injured person goes home. Changes in personality and emotions are often more challenging to the family and caregivers than physical problems. You may find yourself wondering, "Who is this person?" This kind of thought may lead you to feel scared or guilty. It is important to remember that these feelings are normal. There is no right or wrong way to feel when someone you love gets hurt.

You may ask yourself "How can I live with a stranger?" Here are a number of things to think about that might help:

- Realize that not everything has changed and try to recognize the good qualities that are still there. It is natural to focus on the things you don't like. Try to focus on the positive, too.
- Change after injury is ongoing. The behaviors you see now may change over the next few weeks or months. Recognize the injured person's ability to change for the better. Point out what

you see and like.
- Sometimes the injured person acts differently because he or she is treated differently by others. You may be treating this person differently, too. For example, you may be treating your spouse like a child, and this may be making him or her angry.
- Try to do some of the things you used to enjoy doing together. Try taking a walk, seeing a movie, or visiting friends.
- Most of all, try to be patient. It takes time to adapt to changes. Also, not all of the changes you notice now are permanent.

HOW MAY THE ROLES IN OUR FAMILY CHANGE?

Brain injury happens to the whole family. Sometimes it can take family members a long time to recognize the effects of brain injury on the family. It is common for family members and friends to take on additional responsibilities related to caring for the injured person. Some family members may begin to take on responsibilities or roles held by the injured person. It can be especially overwhelming when caregivers are performing their own responsibilities as well as those typically taken care of by the patient. In addition, family members or friends may need to help the injured person get to and from appointments, may have to take on additional household, financial, and childcare responsibilities, and may have to give up their own work responsibilities. Families may experience a reduction in income because the injured person is no longer able to work, and additional expenses may arise from medical bills. While these types of problems do not happen to all patients and their families, when they do happen, they may not be realized until later when the patient returns home.

The way the injured person interacts with others can be different, leading to changes in emotional intimacy. Sometimes this change can be significant enough that the spouse or significant other of the injured person may begin to feel lonely or alone and may grieve for the relationship they had with the patient before the injury happened. This may be a good time to start new routines and new traditions. Find new activities and interests that you can share together to help rebuild some of the closeness you felt before. This may take some time, so try to be patient and ask for help when you need it.

In the first few days and weeks after brain injury, the patient and family may receive many visitors and offers of help. These offers may even feel overwhelming at times. After weeks or months, the situation may change and the person with brain injury and their family may begin to feel isolated. Sometimes visitors stop coming and people stop offering help. Sometimes the person with injury and his or her family stop asking for help, even when they need it. In fact, the weeks and months after returning home may be the time when families need the most help. Many people are uncomfortable asking for help because they might feel that others do not really want to help or may be too busy to help. They may feel that they have already asked for help too many times and that others may be sick of their asking. They may feel that asking for help is a sign of weakness or an admission that they cannot handle things on their own. It may be helpful to realize that asking for help may not be as negative as you think. It lets people know how you are doing and provides an opportunity to continue relationships with people who care about you. It also shows recognition of limitations and allows an opportunity to reduce frustration and more effectively carry out many responsibilities. Try to remember that people who offer help care about you.

WHAT CAN I DO TO HELP MY FAMILY MEMBER?

The family is an important part of the rehabilitation and recovery process. In fact, it is important to remember that the family is part of the rehabilitation team. Research shows that a supportive family has a big impact on the successful recovery of people with brain injuries. Many brain injury survivors need help and motivation when they go home. Friends and family members play a big role by supporting them in doing everyday tasks, remembering to follow recommendations from their therapists, providing transportation, and many other things.

It is also important to know when to step back and let your loved one do things for himself or herself. It might be hard to know when to help and when to step back. It might also be hard to know the right things to do to help your loved one recover as much as possible. Be sure to ask for help in these areas before leaving the hospital. Below are some suggestions for ways that you might be able to help your loved one.

To help with specific physical problems after brain injury see the suggestions in Chapter 5. Be sure to talk with the patient's therapists about how he is doing and what skills he is working on. Go to family conferences and family training sessions to learn as much as you can. Ask the therapists for recommendations about what you can do to help your loved one get better in this area. If the patient cannot sit, stand, or walk alone, you might ask the therapists or doctors how to help the patient transfer or get in and out of the bed or a chair safely. If the patient is walking and needs help with balance, ask the therapists how closely you need to watch, and if there are certain areas or situations where more help is needed. For instance, the patient may need more help on stairs or uneven surfaces than he or she does on a flat, level surface. The best thing you can do is to observe the patient during his or her therapy so that you understand what he or she can and cannot do and what kind of help is needed.

To help with specific cognitive problems after brain injury, see the suggestions in Chapter 6. It may also be helpful to meet with the patient's speech therapist and neuropsychologist to get more information about the types of cognitive problems he or she may be experiencing. The speech therapist and neuropsychologist can give you very specific recommendations for what to do to help the patient with memory problems or any other cognitive problems being experienced.

To help with emotional and behavioral changes after brain injury, see the suggestions in Chapter 7. It is important to remember that these changes are caused by the brain injury and that the patient is not behaving this way on purpose. You may feel angry or embarrassed about these behaviors. Try to remember that these behaviors will change over time as the patient recovers. Relationships are important for everyone. Everyone needs to feel loved and supported. After brain injury, many people feel like no one understands them or what they are going through. They may feel isolated and alone. Talking with the patient and being there for him or her may help one to feel less lonely and more understood. Even if the patient cannot talk or does not know where he or she is, having a familiar face or voice may help him or her to feel safe and comfortable.

WHAT CAN I DO TO HELP MYSELF?

As hard as it may be, try to have patience. Brain injury brings on many sudden changes. Several months after the injury, things seem to move much more slowly, especially when waiting to get appointments, to hear about disability benefits, or to find out test results. One may find comfort in knowing that patience is a skill that can be relearned after brain injury. Take slow deep breaths, count to ten, or focus on improvements, and encourage the brain-injured person to do the same thing. Try to keep in mind that neurological problems are very different from other kinds of health problems, and that getting better can take months or years. Getting irritated with slow progress can make one feel discouraged, and maybe even worse than that. It can push away the people whose help and support are most needed.

Remember that success is relative. Judging the person with the injury by comparing him or her to how he or she was before the injury can bring on disappointment and make frustration worse. Instead, look at the progress that has been made since your family member was injured, and encourage the injured person to do the same thing.

Monitor and manage your stress level. A little stress is a normal part of life, but too much stress has a negative effect on health, ability to do things well, and relationships with others. The first step in controlling stress is recognizing it. When faced with many responsibilities, one may only think about how much there is to be done, how little time there is to do it, and the bad things that will happen if they are not finished. By monitoring stress levels, one can better control his or her actions, feelings, and quality of life.

Once the signs of stress are recognized, it is important to take steps to cope with stress effectively. Below are some ideas that have helped others:

- Take breaks often. Realize that most family members do not give themselves enough rest, and that working harder does not necessarily mean accomplishing more. Take several short breaks each day, even if it is for only 10 minutes.
- Make a list of things that you need to do in the short- and long-term, and set priorities. Start with the top priority and work your way down, realizing that you can only do one or two things at a time effectively. Regularly review your progress to help you keep a more positive perspective. Don't forget that activities related to helping yourself, like getting rest, can also be important priorities, and learn to recognize the difference between what you "have to" do and what you "want to" do.

- Set reasonable expectations and goals. Recognize your limitations and avoid letting people pressure you into taking on more than you can handle.
- Learn and use negotiation skills. Realize that few of your responsibilities are non-negotiable. With coworkers and other family members, negotiate timelines and the amount of responsibilities you agree to take on. If you are afraid of negotiating, practice by rehearsing in your head or in front of a mirror. Balance your wish to please others with your knowledge of what you must do in order to succeed.
- Tell yourself things that help you feel better. "I'm a good person, and I'm doing the best that I can." "We've really come a long way since she was injured." "I can count on my family, friends, and faith to help me get through this."
- Ask for help. In the first days and weeks after the injury, the family may get many offers for help. Weeks or months later, the situation may change. Many family members often feel increased isolation from their extended family and friends. Sometimes people stop offering help, and sometimes the injured person's family members avoid asking for help. Seek help from the people who have offered. Recognize that everyone needs help sometimes, and remember that it is better to ask for help early on rather than when things are coming to a crisis level. Your family member's brain injury has left you and your family with disadvantages. Asking for others' help may be the only way to effectively carry out your responsibilities, meet your personal needs, and make your family stronger.
- Utilize the resources available at your hospital and in your community by asking for assistance from your family member's nurse manager, psychologist, case manager, or social worker, or anyone else on his or her treatment team.
- Try to maintain a sense of humor. A good laugh, even when times are tough, can help you deal with the stress you are facing.
- Participate in a support group. There really is strength in numbers.
- Learn and use relaxation techniques. Listen to soothing music, take a walk, or talk to someone you feel comfortable with. Or practice some of these exercises:
  - Focused breathing. When you are upset or stressed, your breathing becomes shallow and quick. Taking full breaths relax-

es your body. Try lying down comfortably on your back and placing your hands just below your belly button. Close your eyes and
imagine a balloon resting inside your abdomen. Inhale fully and
imagine that the balloon is filling with air. Then exhale slowly,
imagining the balloon collapsing and all your stress leaving your
body. Once you get the hang of it, you can do this exercise sitting or even standing.

- Muscle tensing and relaxing. This exercise helps you notice the difference between the way your body feels when you are tense and
the way it feels when you are relaxed. Begin with curling and tensing your toes as you breathe in and then relaxing them as you
breathe out, noticing the difference in tension as you relax. Repeat
this exercise with other body parts, moving your way up the body.

- Visual imagery. Lie down or sit in a quiet, comfortable place and
imagine yourself in a place where you feel relaxed and calm.
This can be a place that you have been before or a place that you
have always imagined would make you feel relaxed. For example, you can imagine yourself on a beach, restfully lying in the
sand. Try to use all your senses to imagine the feel of the sunshine on your body, the sound of the water, the smells of saltwa-
ter, and the visual beauty of a colorful sunset. If a beach does not
seem relaxing to you, pick another place.

• Get professional help. If things begin to feel out of control and the
tips listed above are no longer helping, it may be time to seek professional help from a social worker or psychologist. This is particularly true if feelings of depression, sadness, or worry begin to interfere with your ability to care for yourself or your loved one.
Warning signs include trouble sleeping (or excessive sleeping), loss
of appetite (or increased appetite), decreased energy and motivation, loss of interest in activities that you used to enjoy, loss of interest in social activities, irritability, thoughts of death or harming
yourself. If you begin to feel this way, get in touch with the treatment team's psychologist, physician, or social worker for a referral.

WHAT SHOULD WE TELL THE CHILDREN?

When a friend or relative has had a brain injury, it is difficult to understand what has happened, how to help, and how to cope. This is true for

adults, and even more so for children. This is especially true when the child was close to the injured person. Children may be scared and confused by the changes they see in this person, and they may be even more scared by the loss of security if this person is their parent or caretaker. Adults often do not know how or when to explain injuries to children. It is also difficult to know when to bring children to the hospital and how to talk to them about what they see and feel after they see a loved one who has been injured. There are no specific ways to handle this, and each child will deal with the situation in his or her own way.

A good rule of thumb is to prepare the children for what has happened by explaining the situation in terms they can understand and by telling them what to expect before they visit the patient in the hospital. When explaining a brain injury to children, it might be helpful to provide an analogy that they can understand. For instance, you can tell them that a brain injury is different from other injuries, and that while broken bones can heal completely, the brain is different. Prepare children for what types of changes to expect, whether they are physical, emotional, or cognitive. It should be explained that the injured person may be very tired, may have difficulty walking, and may act differently than he or she did before. Explain that he or she might say or do things that are strange, and he or she may get angry more easily. Explain to them that these changes will get better over time but no one can say for sure how long it will take to get better.

When planning the first visit, wait until both the children and patient are ready. Children should never be forced or pressured to visit if they are not ready. Phone calls are a good alternative in the beginning until the child and patient feel ready for a face-to-face visit. It may be good to postpone phone calls and visits if the patient is extremely agitated or confused and behaving inappropriately, particularly for younger children who may not understand what is happening. Visits should be planned for times during the day when the patient is the most alert, relaxed, and cooperative. Try not to plan a visit after a tiring therapy session that may have upset or frustrated the patient.

Initial visits should be kept short, and efforts should be made to be with the children after the visit to discuss anything that upset them or any questions they may have. It is important to realize that children process things at their own rate and may not want to discuss what they are feeling. They may not even understand what they are feeling. The best thing to do is to be available when the children are ready to talk and let them know that there is someone they can talk to and ask questions if they would like. You can also enlist the treatment team's psychologist, doctor, or social worker to set up a special family meeting to provide information and answer questions.

Later, when preparing the children for the future, it might be helpful to tell them that over time there may be some things that the injured person cannot do anymore, like playing ball or riding a bike. You can also tell them that some people who have had a brain injury have problems for the rest of their lives, but they still can feel better and learn new ways to do things.

Explaining these things to the children may help them understand what has happened to their loved one. Children usually feel better and are less scared when they understand what is happening. Talking about the injury also lets them know it is all right for them to talk to you about it. If the injured person is a parent, talk with the child about who will be taking care of them and who they can go to for help and comfort.

The National Resource Center has published a book that helps teach children ages 6 to 14 about brain injury and its effects. If you are interested in purchasing the book, contact the National Resource Center to request a catalog at 804-828-9055.

KEY POINTS

- Brain injury affects the family as much as the person who had the brain injury, and the family is an important member of the rehabilitation team.
- Be sure to work with the therapists and doctors so that you know the best ways to help the person with brain injury.
- Sometimes changes in a person's behavior and personality, after he or she has had a brain injury, can be the most stressful for families. Many of these changes may not be noticeable until after going home from the hospital.
- It is as important for caregivers to take care of themselves as it is to take care of the person with brain injury. Learning to recognize when one is feeling stressed or overwhelmed, and finding ways to cope with those feelings, will be essential.
- Don't be afraid to ask for help.

—11—
SUBSTANCE ABUSE AND BRAIN INJURY

WILLIAM GARMOE

No, I never drink alcohol. . . . I only drink beer, you know, like a six-pack after work. —Anonymous

The purpose of this chapter is to address issues related to alcohol and other substance abuse concerns as they relate to traumatic brain injury. This chapter will review information about how alcohol and illicit drugs contribute to brain injuries and will give practical suggestions on what can be done about these problems during recovery. For purposes of simplicity, the term, "substance abuse," will be used throughout the chapter to refer to both alcohol and other drug abuse.

This chapter is relevant to individuals with a history of alcohol or other substance abuse before brain injury. It also applies to people who develop such problems in the years following injury. Also, many individuals engage in what may be termed "risky drinking," which may not meet formal criteria for a disorder but put the person at risk for further injury.

The U. S. Centers for Disease Control (CDC) and others report that alcohol misuse is the greatest risk factor contributing to serious injuries in the United States (Maier, 2005). It is also well documented in studies that alcohol and illicit drugs are major problems in individuals who suffer brain injury. Many professionals make the strong point that alcohol and other drug use are the biggest risk factors for brain injury, especially in adolescents and young adults. A consistent finding is that approximately 30% to 50% of individuals admitted to hospitals with traumatic brain injury (TBI) test positive for alcohol at the time. Research studies at the National Rehabilitation Hospital (NRH) document that

60% to 70% of patients admitted to the TBI treatment program have a positive diagnosis for alcohol abuse.

WHAT IS SUBSTANCE ABUSE?

Substance abuse involves an ongoing pattern of alcohol or other drug use that causes significant emotional distress or interferes with functioning in important life areas. Impaired functioning may involve failure to fulfill major responsibilities, such as keeping a job, attending school, parenting, etc. It may also involve using substances in risky situations, such as when driving or operating machines, getting into legal trouble, and continuing to use alcohol or other drugs in spite of negative effects in life.

An important point to recognize is that substance abuse is not determined entirely by the amount a person is using. The emphasis is on the impact the substance use is having on an individual's life functioning. The most familiar scenario is the individual who drinks alcohol or uses some other drug regularly and excessively, causing great interference in his or her life. Substance abuse is also present if an individual uses alcohol or some other drug occasionally, but in a way that causes major problems. One example of this kind of abuse would include binge drinking. Another would involve a person who engages in risky drinking or drug use; in other words, they may not use the substance every day or even binge, but they put themselves or others at risk when they do it. The adolescent or young adult who "only" drinks once or twice a month, but when he or she gets intoxicated and drives home, may meet criteria for having a substance abuse problem.

Another important point to recognize is that the definition of substance abuse does not only apply to alcohol and illegal drugs. Substance abuse can be diagnosed if an individual is misusing prescription or over-the-counter medications. It also applies when individuals are engaged in activities, such as sniffing glue, huffing, or mixing two legal substances (e.g., alcohol and a prescribed medication) to obtain an altered mental state. Parents should recognize that some of the substances most commonly abused by teenagers are readily available in the home (e.g., inhaling spray paint and other solvents, medications prescribed to others in the home, etc.).

Much less is known about the level of involvement of other drugs, illicit substances, as well as prescription or over-the-counter medicines, as contributing factors to brain injury. Studies at NRH indicate that approximately 30% of patients admitted with a diagnosis of TBI acknowledge illicit drug use. Of course, many individuals who abuse alcohol also use illicit drugs or misuse legal substances such as pain medications.

IMPACT ON RECOVERY

The effects of substance abuse do not end at the time of injury because it creates many potential complications for survival and recovery. Some of these complications include:

- Withdrawal symptoms during the acute trauma care period
- Other medical complications that interfere with survival and recovery
- Longer duration of periods of agitation during recovery
- More severe neuropathological changes in the brain
- Lower scores on cognitive tests at time of discharge from the hospital
- Contribution to long-term adjustment issues

Many families hope that the brain injury has "cured" the individual's substance abuse problem. Part of this hope is that the person with brain injury will either realize the damage he or she was doing or will lose the desire for alcohol or other drug. While this is an understandable hope, it usually is not realistic. When substance abuse in survivors of brain injury is not detected or is ignored, many problems are likely to develop. One of the most obvious is that the person may return to substance use. Research has shown that for individuals with a pre-injury history of substance abuse, a sizable number return to using substances in the two years following injury. Return to substance use is problematic for many reasons. First, it increases the risk for further damage to the brain. Second, it increases the risk for additional brain injuries or other accidents. Third, alcohol and other drugs often have a stronger effect on the person recovering from a brain injury.

There are other important reasons not to ignore a substance abuse problem, even if the person is still in the hospital or is home but not drinking or using another drug. Untreated substance abuse problems very often interfere with an individual's motivation to work hard in rehabilitation and persevere when things get difficult. Substance abuse represents a way of coping with the world, although it is an unhealthy one. Long-term abstinence almost always requires learning new and healthy ways of coping with stress and emotions. If a substance abuse problem is ignored, the individual will likely never have the opportunity to learn better ways to cope, and will be more likely to start using drugs again. Additionally, substance abuse problems often occur together with other psychiatric illnesses, such as depression or anxiety. Sometimes the substance use is a way to self-treat, or self-medicate, the psychiatric illness. When substance abuse is recognized and addressed, other illnesses can also be treated, which will boost recovery from brain injury. Rebuilding life following brain injury is remarkably challenging. The person who suffered a brain injury needs every tool available to help recover.

The person with brain injury often does not experience urges or cravings for alcohol or other drugs while still in the hospital. This situation can build false comfort in family members, who understandably hope that the problem will not return. Unfortunately, once a person leaves the hospital, he or she returns to the real world with stresses as well as many reminders and cues about substance use. For many individuals, it is not until one returns home that he or she fully realizes that he or she cannot easily return to work, school, and other activities. During this challenging period, urges for alcohol or other drugs often return. Finally, sometimes family members or friends offer alcohol or drugs to the person who has returned home following brain injury. If the problem has never been discussed, it is more likely that the person will say yes when it is offered.

ADDRESSING THE PROBLEM

Thorough screening is essential for possible substance abuse problems among persons with brain injury. This screening should be done as early in the recovery process as possible. Several sources of information are used to screen for problems with alcohol or other drugs. These include:
- A clinical assessment conducted by the physician, psychologist, or social worker on the team. This type of assessment may involve the use of structured rating scales or questionnaires, though such instruments sometimes are too complicated for someone with significant cognitive problems

- Review of hospital records that may show evidence of substance abuse
- Discussions with family members about the person's substance use patterns

Family members sometimes feel a need to keep certain things private as a way of protecting the person recovering from brain injury. Families may not be sure whether they can trust the treatment team with sensitive information. Overall, it is best for the person with brain injury not to hide a substance abuse problem. Remember, unidentified substance abuse problems have a negative effect on recovery. Honesty about drinking or using drugs will give the person the opportunity to rebuild his or her life.

One may feel a wide range of emotions about having to talk about substance abuse problems. The individual with a brain injury may feel defensive, angry, or embarrassed about the problem and wish to avoid it or hope that it will just go away. Family members may feel similar emotions. Among family members, emotions may be further complicated because they want to be supportive of the individual with brain injury, but at the same time they feel sad and angry about his or her behavior and the impact it has had on the family and friends. Perhaps the family did not know about the substance abuse problem until the medical team at the trauma hospital told them about the toxicology tests or other information that the clinical team found to indicate the individual had a problem. In this case, family and friends may also be feeling embarrassed, humiliated, guilty, or demoralized. It is important to know that these are normal emotional reactions and it is perfectly okay to have them. It is not good, however, to let these feelings make one avoid talking about the substance abuse problems. Difficult emotions can be dealt with, but only if they are discussed in the right setting. The substance abuse problem needs to be addressed.

INTERVENTIONS

Addressing a substance abuse problem in a person recovering from brain injury starts with communication. It is important that family members find ways to talk with the person recovering from brain injury about his or her problem. It is not unkind to bring up the problem. Substance abuse is a major health problem, and just as with other conditions such as a heart attack or cancer, it needs to be acknowledged and discussed. Of course there needs to be sensitivity about when to discuss the problem and the person's cognitive status needs to be taken into account. The harm from not discussing the problem is much worse than the hurt feelings that may result when it is discussed. The psychologist or social worker on the team may be able to help family members become more comfortable talking to the recovering person about substance abuse concerns.

Early in recovery, treatment of substance abuse problems often involves very basic education and simple statements about the importance of not returning to alcohol or other drugs. As the person's cognitive abilities improve, treatment can become more active. Treatment of substance abuse problems with individuals recovering from brain injury has many similarities to programs found in the community. Alcoholics Anonymous (AA) and Narcotics Anonymous (NA) type groups are often used, and those that include others who have suffered brain injuries or other brain syndromes can be particularly effective.

Individual treatment in the hospital and after discharge may be provided by a psychologist or social worker on the rehabilitation team. These professionals will have detailed understanding of the interaction of brain injury and substance use. Specialized programs in the community may also be good resources. When the problem is severe, the team may recommend that the person recovering from brain injury be discharged directly from the hospital into a residential substance abuse program. Medications may be used, but usually are not prescribed to directly address urges for alcohol or other drugs. Rather, medications are usually used to treat behavioral difficulties that increase the risk for substance use (such as agitation, distractibility, etc.) and psychiatric problems (such as depression or anxiety).

Special considerations need to be taken into account when providing substance abuse treatment to individuals recovering from brain injury. Because of the cognitive deficits that result from brain injury, the individual may not comprehend pamphlets and other written materials. Substance abuse treatment often involves significant amounts of reading, which can overwhelm the person with brain injury and unintentionally have a negative effect on motivation. Materials need to be simplified and often reduced to short, direct sentences. Individuals recovering from brain injury are more likely to forget what was learned and have difficulties with mental flexibility, which can limit how well they grasp and incorporate new ideas and principles. Individuals recovering from brain injury may also have difficulty sustaining attention for the length of time many self-help and treatment groups last. A further point to consider is that substance abuse treatment often relies heavily on confrontation by others. Individuals with brain injury who are prone to agitation, may be provoked by confrontation that is too intense. It will be important that those providing the substance abuse treatment know about the brain injury and the need to adapt techniques and written materials so the individual with brain injury can get the full benefit.

Special consideration also needs to be made for individuals with significant self-awareness deficits and motivational problems following brain injury. The individual with impaired self-awareness may appear to be in deep psychological denial about a substance abuse problem. Impaired self-awareness and conditions of reduced motivation caused by the brain injury may be mistaken as deep psychological denial and refusal to participate. The result will be frustration for everyone involved. If problems with self-awareness are severe, the focus of substance abuse treatment will need to be on controlling access to alcohol and other drugs as much as on education and therapy.

LOOKING INTO THE FUTURE

For individuals with a history of alcohol or other drug abuse prior to brain injury, the only prudent recommendation is that they commit to completely abstain from substance use for the remainder of their lifetime. On one level this is a parsimonious recommendation. First, there are no conditions under which return to illicit/illegal drug use can be condoned. Second, very few, if any, individuals with a history of alcohol abuse can return to drinking safely. This point is doubly important when applied to individuals recovering from brain injury. Quite simply, the risks for further brain damage and further life problems are too great to even consider that drinking could be realistic.

This point cannot be over-emphasized. Individuals in denial of their substance abuse problems look for reasons to justify their alcohol or other drug use, including not being honest with physicians and mental health workers about the amount they consume. This chapter is unequivocal in emphasizing that, if a person has a history of substance abuse, he or she should never consume alcohol or use drugs again. Period.

But many individuals who suffer brain injury do not have a history of alcohol abuse. Should they also be advised not to ever drink alcohol again? This is a complicated matter. On the one hand, there are risks associated with alcohol use even for individuals with no substance abuse history. Even modest amounts of alcohol may have a negative effect on thinking, memory, and coordination, all of which may increase the risk for falls or other accidents. Many of the medications prescribed for individuals with brain injury can be harmful if mixed with alcohol. Some individuals will have an increased risk for seizures from drinking. Additionally, consequences of brain injury can increase the risk of developing alcohol abuse, even in individuals who have no prior history of such problems. Individuals with brain injury have a higher risk for depression and anxiety in the years following injury. Many individuals with brain injury also suffer loss of important life roles, decrease in the number of close and supportive relationships, experience social isolation, loneliness, and boredom, all of which can be risk factors for alcohol abuse.

Alternatively, individuals recovering from brain injury want, and deserve, to return to as many normal adult roles and responsibilities as possible. Alcohol is part of many normal adult social activities in our society. Most adults are responsible in their drinking patterns, so is it fair to expect a person with a brain injury not to drink any alcohol, even if they are doing very well in their recovery? There is no easy answer to this question, but some guidelines may be helpful. First, the most conservative and safe solution would be for the person with brain injury to abstain from alcohol use entirely. Second, if an individual with brain injury does want to resume responsible alcohol use, he or she should first discuss it thoroughly with his or her physician, psychologist and family members. This may seem like an unfair standard, but if family members or the physician or psychologist/social worker think it is a bad idea, it would probably be best to accept it and not drink. Third, if responsible alcohol use is resumed, the person with brain injury needs to wait until his or her physician is comfortable with how far post-injury he or she is, and only modest amounts should ever be consumed. It is also critical that alcohol only be consumed in very safe situations (e.g., no driving, potentially unsafe activities, etc.) Finally, the person with brain injury needs to be open to the possibility that, if there are negative consequences to alcohol use, others may see them before he or she does. A spirit of openness to feedback is very important.

KEY POINTS

- Substance abuse after a brain injury puts one at significant risk for another brain injury.
- Substance abuse after brain injury can worsen mood disorders, such as depression.
- People with a history of alcohol abuse have lower scores on cognitive testing at time of discharge from the hospital.
- After a brain injury, one should consult with a physician and/or psychologist before consuming alcohol.

12

BRAIN INJURY AND SEXUALITY

PENNY WOLFE
NEEPA SHAH
LAUREN ZIMMERMAN

*I was afraid and embarrassed to ask my doctor if I would be able to
have sex after my injury. But, I was so happy when my doctor
told me that I would be able to be intimate with my wife again.*
—Anonymous

Sexuality is a normal part of the
human experience. We are social beings and part of that includes the
desire to seek out relationships with others. Sexuality does not just relate
to the physical aspects of sex; it also relates to one's ability to form intimate relationships with others, one's understanding of his or her gender,
and a desire to feel connected to another person. It is important to
remember that individuals who have a brain injury are still social, and
therefore sexual, beings. However, the experience of a traumatic brain
injury may affect one's sexuality for various reasons. Brain injury can
bring about different physical, cognitive, or emotional problems that may
alter one's ability to be in a sexual relationship. It is important to recognize and address these factors throughout the process of rehabilitation.

Changes in sexual functioning following acquired brain injury are
very common and may be caused by several factors. Both persons with
brain injury, and their partners, often have many questions about what
to expect. Unfortunately, not all persons feel comfortable discussing
issues related to sexuality, even with their healthcare professionals. This
chapter is designed to provide an overview of topics related to potential
sex-related issues and what can be done to address them. This chapter
includes information on the following topics:

- The body's response
- Changes in sexual desire
- Changes in roles and relationships
- Is it safe to have sex?
- Self-image
- Emotional Issues
- Decreased social contact or opportunities
- How to get help
- How to discuss sex with a healthcare professional

THE BODY'S RESPONSE

The following sections will provide information about some of the changes that may affect sexuality and/or sexual performance in persons who have suffered a brain injury.

Physical/Sensory-Motor

Depending on the location of the injury within the brain, the effects of traumatic brain injury on sexual function can vary. For example, injury to the sensory-motor strip area of the brain could lead to muscle weakness, reduced coordination, changes in sensation or pain. These physical impairments can sometimes disrupt sexual activity. An injury to the occipital lobe may result in changes in vision or may narrow one's visual field. This type of sensory deficit can usually be compensated for, but may result in difficulties connecting and communicating with a partner on a date or in intimate situations. It is important to become educated about the location of the injury you or your loved one experienced, the expected deficits, and how these deficits can impact everyday functioning, including sexual activity.

Sexual dysfunction is the term used to describe disturbances in one's ability to participate in normal sexual activity. Dysfunction can come about by both primary (physical or organic) or secondary (psychological or social) causes or a combination of both. It is not uncommon for individuals with traumatic brain injury (TBI) to develop sexual dysfunction. Fortunately, many treatment options exist that can help address the causes of sexual dysfunction ranging from the use of medication to participation in psychotherapy. The following will explore some of the most common physiological impairments along with the resulting sexual dysfunctions seen in individuals with brain injuries.

Decreased Arousal

One of the most common effects a brain injury can have on sexual functioning is decreased sexual arousal or "libido." This can be brought about not only from changes to regions in the brain involved in sexual arousal (the limbic system), but also by other factors, such as medication side effects, emotional disturbances such as depression, or even from cognitive deficits such as apathy or confusion. Certain commonly used medications, such as some antidepressants, may result in decreased sexual arousal or difficulty with achieving an erection and/or orgasm. If a person experiences these types of changes, it is essential to speak with one's physician before stopping the medication. The physician can help determine if the sexual changes are caused by medication or are occurring for another reason. Also, if a person with brain injury abruptly stops taking certain medications, he or she is at risk for potentially negative side-effects, such as seizures.

It is important for the individual and the partner to be patient and understanding of reduced arousal, to not place undue pressure or blame on oneself or one's partner, and to find different creative ways to increase arousal or simply enjoy one another's company. While it is more common to experience decreased arousal (hyposexuality), some persons with TBI may experience increased arousal (hypersexuality).

Sexual Responsiveness

Sometimes even when arousal occurs, problems in genital functioning may hinder the act of intimacy. Common problems in men include weakened or absent erection (often referred to as "impotence" or "erectile dysfunction"), premature ejaculation, or the inability to achieve orgasm. Medication is the most widely used treatment of erectile dysfunction. However, use of this medication may sometimes have to be avoided in this population because of side effects, such as increased blood pressure or clotting. Ask your doctor if you are at risk. Problems most commonly seen in women include decreased vaginal lubrication or inability to achieve orgasm. Artificial lubrication, such as KY Jelly™, may be used to treat this condition.

Incontinence

Incontinence is another common physiological effect of brain injury and one that can greatly impact one's ability or desire to engage in sexual activity. Inability to control one's bladder while being intimate with a partner may create embarrassment and can be very distracting. One simple way to help prevent this problem is to limit liquid intake or use the bathroom right before sex. Other tips include using plastic covering on the bed or having cleaning supplies readily available in the event that an accident does occur. Individuals who use a catheter may be able to remove this device right before engaging in sex. Also, men may be able to cover the catheter with a condom or women can tape it to their side in order to prevent it from interfering.

Motor Abilities

As mentioned, one's motor abilities can be compromised as a result of a traumatic brain injury. Motor deficits can include poor coordination, muscle spasticity, balance problems, muscle weakness or paralysis, decreased range of motion, and pain. Conditions such as apraxia (inability to perform voluntary movements on command) or ataxia (jerky, uncoordinated movements) can develop. Limitations in motor abilities can impact one's ability to engage in foreplay or the act of sex or can cause distractions in the process of attempting. It is important for the couple to discuss the reality of the limitation and make efforts to compensate for these difficulties (i.e., use positions that work well for the individual with brain injury or having the non-brain injured partner positioned on top).

Sensory Changes

Being intimate with another person is a very sensory experience that taps into all five of our senses. Deficits in touch, taste, smell, vision, or hearing can detract from the ability to fully experience the presence of another. For example, visual field cuts or neglect are common in those with brain injury and can take away from one's ability to make eye contact, anticipate body posture, or have awareness of the location of another person. Along with taking efforts to correct the sensation that has been affected, partners should discuss ways to play up the senses that are still intact. For instance, someone with a hearing deficit can learn to rely more on nonverbal communication during sex or someone with tactile sensitivity can find alternatives to traditional sexual activities that do not elicit painful or over-stimulating responses.

Cognition

Engaging in sexual activity requires more thought and coordination of different cognitive faculties than one might imagine. The act of foreplay alone requires judgment, initiation, memory, motor sequencing, and mental flexibility. The experience of a brain injury can sometimes leave long-lasting impacts on one's ability to think efficiently and clearly and can impact his or her ability to participate in sexual activity. Cognitive deficits are often the result of injury to the frontal or temporal lobe. The presence of cognitive impairment may not only leave the brain injured person confused and anxious about sex, but can also be challenging for a partner to manage as well.

Communication

Those who experience a brain injury may also develop problems with their speech or their ability to comprehend other's verbal communication. Deficits in speech can affect every aspect of personal communication, including dating, communicating or hearing messages in intimate settings, or being able to understand the needs of another. Nonverbal communication impairment can also pose challenges in these instances. Speech therapists, mental health professionals, and others who work with brain injury survivors in helping to improve language abilities can work toward improving communication in the context of dating and intimacy. Those with communication deficits are encouraged to explore alternative methods of expressing oneself, to be patient with the process, and to seek professional help along the way to help improve needed skills.

Executive Functioning

This area of cognition refers to one's ability to plan, organize, and initiate tasks as well as manage one's reactions and behaviors. Common executive functioning deficits seen in those with brain injury (frontal lobe injury in particular) include disinhibition, poor self-awareness, impulsivity, poor judgment/problem solving, and impaired initiation and motivation. Impaired executive abilities can affect sexuality in several ways. Impulsivity and poor self-awareness may cause someone to make unwanted sexual advances to others or may even lead to them being taken advantage of by others. Poor judgment can contribute to engaging in unhealthy sexual practice, such as not using contraception, or can cause the individual to have difficulty in understanding and responding properly to the behaviors of his or her partner. Difficulties initiating or making advances toward one's partner can create the misperception that one is disinterested in sex. Cognitive deficits in this arena can be very problematic to one's ability to participate in appropriate, mature sexual relations. It is important to have an accurate understanding of the type of executive problem present and how to create compensatory or protective strategies to prevent the exploitation of the injured individual or his or her partner.

Memory

Memory processes encapsulate the abilities to attend to, learn, manipulate, and/or recall information. If there is impairment in any of these aspects of memory, engaging in conversation, foreplay, or sexual activity can be compromised. For example, poor attention may make it difficulty to concentrate on conversation with a partner. Impaired immediate memory may impact ability to remember and follow directions or requests by one's partner. Poor delayed memory may cause forgetfulness of routine or the learned preferences of a partner.

Emotional Status

Changes in emotional states, mood, and self-image can also occur in those with traumatic brain injury. Examples include the onset of depression, poor self-esteem, lack of motivation, and even agitation or mania. Emotional problems can emerge as the result of physical and chemical changes to the brain, or they may come about as a result of difficulty coping and adapting to life after injury. Changes in the way you feel about yourself, about your environment, and about others can influence intimate relationships with partners or may interfere with dating. For example, depression is often a leading cause of sexual dysfunction in both men and women. It is important to address and talk about these feelings with someone you can trust. The use of medication or participation in counseling may also help. The following list describes the role that many common emotional problems may play in relationships and expression of sexuality:

- Depression
- Anxiety and agitation
- Apathy, lack of emotion
- Mania, excess emotion

When sexual activity is truly not an option because of physical, cognitive, or emotional deficits, couples are always encouraged to explore alternatives for intimacy such as massage, hugging, talking, or your own creative way to celebrate your loved one's company!

In addition to changes that may occur in the genital area, there may be changes in other parts of the body that affect a person's ability to perform sexual activity. For example, a man who has weakness on one side of his body will likely have difficulty or find it impossible to have sex in the traditional missionary position (man on top). Therefore, it is important to be creative and try different positions.

IS IT SAFE TO HAVE SEX?

Several factors should be considered when determining if it is safe to return to sexual activity following brain injury. First and foremost, one should have an open discussion with the physician in charge of care.

There may be medical issues that need to be considered before one returns to sexual activity. For instance, a person with a brain injury may also have orthopedic injuries (e.g., broken bones, dislocated joints, etc.) that could be further injured if one engages in sexual activity before full healing has taken place. Problems with high blood pressure, open wounds, or infections may also be reason for one to speak with a physician prior to engaging in sexual activity. Another issue one might need to consider is that the person with brain injury may be too confused or disoriented to fully consent to having a sexual relationship.

Following brain injury, women are still able to become pregnant and men are able to impregnate women. Therefore, contraceptive use (such a condoms or birth control pills) will need to be used to prevent an unwanted pregnancy.

CHANGES IN SELF-IMAGE

Sexuality is characterized by a quality or state of being distinguished by sex and is associated with preparedness for engaging in sexual activity, sexual character, and recognition of sexual matters. It has more to do with who one is as a human being in your relationships and interactions more that the act of sex itself. Sexuality is influenced by how one perceives himself or herself as a sexual being or self-image. Self-image is how one sees himself or herself, what he or she thinks he or she looks like, what kind of person he or she thinks he or she is, how one believes others see him or her, and how much one likes himself or herself. Self-esteem is how one feels about oneself, how one feels about what he or she looks like, and how one feels about what kind of person he or she is. For example, if one sees himself or herself as undesirable or having a poor self-image, then one may not feel confident about his or her sexuality.

After a brain injury, the physiological changes to the brain often result in impaired cognitive processing of feelings, thoughts, and self-awareness. One may also experience changes in how he or she relates to others or have personality or behavioral changes. These changes may influence one's self-image, feelings about their sexuality, and lead to disruptions in social relationships. Another consequence of brain injury, which is often the most noticeable change, is in physical appearance. Deficits in motor function or the ability to walk can lead to feelings of inadequacy as well.

Early in the rehabilitation process, a person with a brain injury is often told what to do and when to do it by his doctors, nurses, therapists and family. From the beginning the individual may feel defined by the way others treat him or her, speak to him or her, or do things for him or her. He or she may feel, whether consciously or unconsciously, as though his or her decision-making abilities and sense of control have been taken away, which can lead to decreased confidence and self-worth. Once out of the hospital setting, an ongoing poor self-image can result in emotional or behavioral problems and continued difficulty in relationships and social settings. Withdrawing from social interaction or attention-seeking behavior can persist in persons with a brain injury. If problems of this nature were present prior to the injury, then these pre-existing behaviors may be difficult to improve upon. They may be further complicated by the physical, cognitive, and behavioral deficits from the head injury. Therefore, it is essential to pay attention to these matters of self-perception and image as a person starts to regain his or her self-awareness, if not before.

It is important to treat a person with a brain injury with age-appropriate, realistic, and factual feedback as observed. Laughing at, or explaining away, a mistake or unusual comment may not be the most effective way to help the person with the brain injury. Giving feedback by saying, "actually the date today is ____ and I believe you are thinking about what happened last month" may reorient someone while maintaining the dignity of the person with the brain injury. This strategy is important when dealing with sexuality as well.

After a brain injury it is not uncommon for a person to go through a period of self-stimulatory behaviors such as masturbation. In the early stages of recovery, it is necessary to allow for self-exploration with privacy and safety in mind. In addition, as speech improves, a person with brain injury may show disinhibited behavior, such as cursing or making sexual references. It can be uncomfortable or embarrassing for one's family or caregivers. It is also important to remember that adolescents who have had a brain injury may have been in the sexual experimental phase of their development at the time of injury. Therefore this behavior may be appropriate for their developmental recovery and age-appropriate sexual education presented in a clear and concise method would be beneficial.

SOCIAL CONTACT/DECREASED OPPORTUNITY

As the person with the brain injury recovers and returns to the community, he or she may encounter situations outside of the controlled and structured environment of the hospital. These situations may cause some regression, feelings of frustration, and sense of failure. He or she may become more isolated, lonely, irritable, and hostile. As these feelings progress, sexual desire or interest may wane, further isolating them and causing the person to feel depressed. These feelings can also affect the healthy partner of a brain-injured individual. It is normal for a partner to be conflicted and apprehensive about resuming a sexual relationship. Seeing a loved one in a childlike state, in an angry agitated phase, or with a physical disability is a difficult ordeal. Dealing with guilt, anger, loss, and/or frustration can lead to feelings of resentment or disinterest in a sexual relationship. It is important too that both partners communicate with each other to discuss interest or concerns about resuming intimacy in a relationship. Both people should be comfortable and willing to explore options if there are physical, cognitive, or behavioral limitations to consider. Certain physical deficits can pose a challenge when attempting to return to a sexual relationships. Hemiplegia, hemisensory deficits, poor trunk control or balance, and ataxia are just some of the physical limitations that can be addressed by your occupational therapist who can suggest some positions, equipment, or techniques that will allow for a more safe experience for both partners. Even medical complications, such as seizures, should be a consideration. Education on contraception, safe sex practices, sexually transmitted diseases (STDs), adjustment to disability, and appropriate behavior and respect for your partner should also be initiated in therapy sessions. Many healthcare professionals, such as your doctor, nurse, occupational therapist, psychologist, or sex therapist, can assist or give you references for more information. It is important to seek out the individuals with whom you feel most comfortable discussing this. If they are unable to help you, they can guide you to the most appropriate person. Establishing this professional support system is beneficial for ongoing guidance, especially if you are planning to get pregnant.

For the single person who has a brain injury, resuming a social life and finding opportunities for sexual contact can be challenging. Often times it will be family members who help with finding social groups or outlets. This effort requires a lot of time and dedication and can be frustrating when boundaries between roles are blurred. Conflict may occur when family members take on the role of trying to provide appropriate social outlets for the brain-injured person. For example, a parent who wants to help a brain injured son improve his social life by dating may also feel that he or she has to be a chaperone or protector.

To address some of these areas of sexuality, one may want to consider seeking out peer support groups, counseling, or structured programs that focus on these areas. These types of groups or counseling programs may focus on issues, such as appearance and hygiene, dealing with discrimination, marketing oneself, contraception, sexual dysfunction, medications and side effects, and being realistic about oneself. Not only the return to an active and responsible sex life, but also the establishment of one's sexuality or sexual identity, are large parts of rebuilding self-esteem, image, and societal reintegration.

Changes in Roles and Relationships

As expected, the experience of a traumatic brain injury not only affects the individual but also his or her partner in many aspects of daily living. Changes in sexual functioning, desire, or ability brought about by the brain injury can be challenging for both the affected individual and his or her partner. It is important to recognize and address the experiences of the healthy partner as well as the injured individual. The healthy partner's experience is unique in that his or her ability, interest, and capacity have not changed directly because of the injury. However, interest may change as a result of taking on new caretaking roles or in part with attempts to adjust to his or her loved one's changes in behavior, physical ability, or cognition. The healthy partner must learn to adapt to the changes that may be present in the partner with a brain injury. This adjustment process is likely to cause frustration, confusion, and sometimes guilt. While such reactions are expected, it is helpful to address these concerns early on to help maintain the relationship and ease the concerns of the brain-injured person and his or her partner. Getting back into a normal sense of life often involved the reintegration of sexual activity so let's take a look at some of the changes that may occur in the relationship and learn how to address them.

The Couple

Engaging in physical intimacy is a normal and healthy way of expressing love and affection for one's partner. Part of the rehabilitation process and road to recovery is restoring this natural element of a relationship. Couples should not ignore the role sex plays in resuming normalcy in relationships because all too often dismissal of this topic can cause rifts between partners and may lead to relationship stress. While many couples resume normal sexual routines, some may need to make adjustments to their sexual repertoire. Necessary changes may include becoming accustomed to decrease (and sometimes increase) in the desire for frequency on behalf of the brain-injured individual. The perception of sex appeal, capacity, or desire may change by either partner following the injury.

It is important to examine the role of sexuality in the context of the couple's life cycle. (Are they young and wanting to reproduce? Are they older and placing emphasis on other parts of their relationship?) Even gender should be examined. (Is the female the caretaker? The injured individual?). It is also necessary to examine the health of the relationship before the onset of injury to determine the role of potential pre-existing problems. Whether a person is in a committed relationship or not will also affect aspects of sexuality. Those who are single and those who are in relationships may face different challenges in restoring healthy sexual functioning.

The Non-Injured Partner or "Caretaker"

One of the most common ways in which the dynamic of relationships change in the context of brain injury is that the healthy partner must often adopt the role of primary caretaker. While, of course, this is a role that partners often willingly and selflessly take on, it is essential for caretakers to still make their own needs a priority and establish appropriate boundaries with the tasks they take on in helping their loved one. Taking on too much of the caretaking responsibility can leave you at risk of burnout and may decrease your interest in relaxing and engaging in pleasurable opportunities. Overextending one's role as a caretaker may limit ability to still serve as a lover and partner. A common boundary that can be blurred that may have consequences on sexual activity is toi-

leting or bathing. For example, if assistance is given in cleaning genitals after urination or excretion, it may sometimes be difficult for
both partners to shift modalities into viewing the genitals as pleas-
ure-producing body parts. There is no shame in using the help of
outside caretakers to assist with these responsibilities. If this is not
feasible, it is possible to set up time schedules or locations for separate activities to keep the sexual bond distinct and sacred.

Furthermore, caretakers may often find themselves in a predica-
ment when it comes to approaching their partner about sex: If they
seek out opportunities for intimacy they may fear coming across as
aggressive or insensitive, but if they avoid opportunities for intimacy, they may fear coming across as cold or disinterested (Rolland,
1994). While each brain-injured person will have different levels of
physical and/or cognitive ability for sex, the healthy partner should
find ways to strike a balance between sensitivity to his or her needs
and the needs of the other. Often it is the tendency of the caretaker
to take on the overprotective role in which he or she may unknowingly treat their loved one as a child or as fragile. If the individual
with brain injury is consenting and able to make decisions, the
healthy partner must learn to treat the brain-injured partner as an
equal and feel free to communicate openly about his or her own
needs. However, if the partner with brain injury does present with
childlike dependency or inappropriate sexual advances, it may be
necessary to set limits in intimate settings.

Changes in sexual desire may also occur in the spouse or partner
of the person with brain injury. Many times the spouse/partner is
required to take on the role of caregiver, which may involve providing personal care. For example, a spouse/partner may have to assist
with tasks such bathing, toileting, changing a diaper, and so forth.
While most spouses/partners adjust to providing this type of assistance, there is also a potential for affecting his or her own desire for
sexual activity with his or her loved one. It is important to recognize
this as a common experience; many spouses/partners have felt the
very same way. These feelings often lead the spouse/partner of a person with brain injury to feel guilty, ashamed, and fearful of being
judged. If this should occur, it is important to be able to talk about it
with a healthcare provider (such as a nurse or doctor) or with a psychologist or counselor.

The Brain-Injured Partner

Not only does the uninjured partner have to integrate the role of care-taker into the relationship, but also the brain-injured partner sometimes has to integrate the role of "patient." Sometimes feelings of guilt or inadequacy can accompany the role of "patient." Frustration may also occur when the individual recovering from a brain injury feels that he or she is not satisfying the other sexually. Those who find themselves experiencing these feelings should feel free to openly communicate with their partners in order to preserve their self-esteem and feelings of worth in the relationship. Often an honest discussion about the adjust-ments each one is making post-injury will foster a sense of connected-ness and can further deepen bonds.

Brain injury survivors may also have to adjust to their new-found lim-itations (physically, cognitively, or emotionally) that may inhibit their ability to participate in what used to feel like an automatic process. Motor limitations may create the need to adopt new techniques or posi-tions when becoming intimate. Cognitive deficits may require the indi-vidual to closely monitor his or her movements and consciously focus on the motor sequencing and steps needed to perform desired activities. Emotional changes may increase or decrease their desire or ability to engage in intimate acts. The confusion and frustration that comes along with these adjustments is often normal and will hopefully improve with time and practice. Again, solid communication with one's partner may help defuse tension or anxiety.

Dating

A high percentage of people that experience brain injuries may not be involved in pre-existing relationships that need to be maintained post-injury. Some may interpret this as a positive, as it may reduce pressure and allow further time for self-improvement. However, others may see this as frustrating, as dating can often be challenging for individuals recovering from brain injury. Regardless of your perspective, each TBI survivor, single or not, is still entitled to desire companionship and inti-macy and should be given opportunities to fulfill these desires (within safe and appropriate limits). Dating can be challenging for someone recovering from brain injury for various reasons (i.e., lack of transportation if driving is not an option, having to explain to others your injury, or even being motivated or having the cognitive skill set needed to engage in proper interactions). When cognitive problems, such as lack of self-awareness or self-control, are present, safety issues can even arise. Individuals with brain injury need to ensure that they are not being put in a situation where they could make unknowingly unwanted advances or where others could possibly take advantage of them.

Sometimes a person with brain injury, one of their caretakers, or healthcare professionals may conclude that dating and/or sexuality activity should be low on the priority list until the individual has an opportunity to further heal and gain more skills that will set them up for success once ready. This advice applies to individuals with partners as well: Survivors of brain injury should feel okay about taking time for oneself and allowing for healing without the distractions of feeling obligated to respond to the needs of others. Once you can work on yourself to be happy with your abilities and who you are, the more likely you are to have successful relationships down the road. One should not underestimate the power of friendship and even of the bonds made in support groups and in therapies in fulfilling the need for human connectivity. Enjoying simple leisure activities and social events can be very rewarding and can serve as a good starting place in the process of recovery. One must also not overlook the fact that sexual pleasure can be achieved independently through masturbation, a natural and healthy way to create feelings of satisfaction and sexual enjoyment.

Tips for Enjoying Sex

Change in functional abilities does not necessarily mean change in ability to give and receive pleasure with one's partner. Sexuality and intimacy can be expressed in a myriad of ways. The limitations brought about by brain injury may likely necessitate the need to think outside the box and explore creative ways to foster closeness and intimacy. First, couples are encouraged to speak openly and honestly about their fears, desires, or concerns. Often, problems can be solved by some old-fashioned communication! Use alternative forms of communicating (i.e., touch or body language) if speech deficits are present. If physical limitations are present, certain positions can be avoided or the healthy partner may choose to take on the more active role (i.e., being on top during missionary sex). If weakness exists on one side of the body, pillows can be used to prop oneself up or reliance on the intact side of the body should be used. When sexual intercourse is not a realistic option, explore alternative forms of intimacy such as massage, kissing, oral sex, or caressing. Make efforts to feel good about oneself by continuing to groom and maintain personal hygiene, set a romantic tone in your bedroom, or even wear something that makes you feel desirable.

When such efforts do not work, professional assistance may be able to provide relief to the frustrated couple, give suggestions for alternative means of sexual expression, and help the couple to make decisions that are healthy and appropriate for their unique circumstance.

How to Discuss Sex with a Healthcare Professional

Will I be able to have sex again? Will my partner be able to perform how he used to? Can I still have children? These questions represent just the tip of the iceberg of concerns individuals affected by TBI and their partners may have about sexual functioning. Questions about this important aspect of life can emerge during inpatient rehabilitation but may often not arise until attempts are made to assimilate into old routines back at home. Unfortunately, many of these questions go unasked due to various reasons, such as level of comfort, personal beliefs, or fear of embarrassment. It is hoped that this message may help encourage those of you who have these questions to speak up: Go ahead and ask! Again, sexuality is a fundamental aspect of human functioning and should be treated as a topic that is fair game for exploration with your healthcare professional. Therapists, doctors, nurses, and others working on rehabilitation teams are trained and able to discuss the questions you may have.

Your entire treatment team is available to discuss aspects of your sexuality. Your physicians and nurses can consult about medication and the physiological aspects of a person's sexual functioning. Consultation with an urologist, one who specializes in the male reproductive system, or a gynecologist, one who specializes in the female reproductive system, can be set up to address concerns about physical ability or fertility. Physical therapists may be able to recommend techniques or positions that can be used to enhance the sexual experience. Occupational therapists help with fine motor skills and restoring activities of daily living, both of which have applicability to sexual activity. Mental health professionals, such as psychologists, can provide supportive therapy, psycho-education about sexuality, and can help to tackle problems with depression or relationships. Often times, difficulties with sexual functioning can subside after issues such as mood, coping with change of abilities, or improved communication occurs.

The benefits of using mental health services deserves further discussion in order to explain what skills can be learned and what issues can be addressed in a therapeutic context. Therapy can be conducted in one-on-one, as a couple, or in a group setting. Based on your level of comfort and goals for treatment, some treatment types may be more appropriate than others. The peer support you receive in a group therapy context can be very helpful in realizing that you are not alone in your struggles. Often, people who have walked a mile in your shoes are best equipped to give you advice. Couples therapy can be very beneficial to a couple in helping to improve lines of communication, to gain a deeper appreciation of each other's partner's needs and concerns, and even to set appropriate boundaries and expectations. Individual therapy can be very useful in addressing overarching issues of depression or anxiety, can help promote acceptance and positive self-esteem, and can even be a good avenue to explore issues of grief and loss of one's abilities. When cognitive problems are present, mental health professionals can help you learn to make good decisions, control impulses, as well as determine what constitutes appropriate sexual activity in efforts to promote and optimize sexual wellness.

KEY POINTS

- Sexuality is a normal part of the human experience.
- Physical, cognitive, and/or emotional changes after a traumatic injury may impact one's sexuality on multiple levels.
- Do feel free to discuss issues related to sexuality, sexual activity, self-image, and relationship issues with a healthcare provider.

——13——

EDUCATION AND VOCATION

SUSAN KAUFFMAN
PENNY WOLFE
MICHAEL YOCHELSON

*We are working together to push past this as a family and get our lives
back in order. While it may be a different, slightly reconfigured life,
I'm highly motivated to make it a rich and rewarding one for all of us.*
—Brian Mosko

People who have sustained a brain
injury can, and do, pursue post-secondary education options. However,
one should take into account an academic setting that will meet the person's individual needs to achieve educational and life goals. The information in this chapter will help prepare students and future students for
successful post-secondary education (college) and assist them in determining if post-secondary education is an appropriate goal.

PLANNING FOR POST-SECONDARY EDUCATION

An important part of setting goals for post-secondary education is determining whether a school is able to meet the needs of the student. Post-secondary education should not be thought of as one modality, but as
many. Post-secondary education does not have to consist of a four-year
college or university, which is how it is often portrayed. Post-secondary
education options can consist of two and four year colleges or universities and/or vocational and career schools. Degrees can also be obtained
through community colleges and associate degree programs.
Community colleges and associate programs often allow the student to

live at home, take lighter course loads, and have flexible academic schedules. Choosing an alternative to a four-year school can also provide a foundation to determine if higher education institutions will be appropriate academic choices in the future. The student should evaluate his or her educational goals to find out if they are appropriate and achievable as new strengths and weaknesses will have to be taken into consideration. The student may wish to discuss this with family members and professionals who know his or her strengths and weaknesses well. Also, the student should find out if the school of choice will be able to assist in meeting educational goals (the specific areas the student wants to study) and what kind of geographical area is preferred (city, suburb, location close to home).

Tips for Researching a School

When researching a post-secondary education option, several tips can be helpful for this process. Making contact with the school's Disability Support Services (DSS) is a good place to start. Disability Support Services assist students with special learning needs. When meeting with a staff member at DSS, find out if the student is an appropriate candidate for the school and, if so, what type of in-service support does the school offer that will assist his or her educational experience. Be sure to ask how accommodations are determined and how flexible the school is in granting them. Also, does the college have faculty and/or administration that understand brain injury and has the school worked with students with brain injury before? What is their success rate? Is the campus accessible for students with physical limitations?

Helpful Facts

Students do not have to inform a post-secondary school of a disability unless academic adjustment services are desired. However, to receive academic adjustments, the student will most likely need to prove his or her disability, which can be done by providing sufficient documentation. Documentation can include medical records, evaluations, date of diagnosis, how the diagnosis was reached, and how the disability affects major life activities and academic performance. Medical and psychological records sometimes contain very personal information that the student may not want to share with the school, so it is important to review the records before submitting them. It is also helpful to provide secondary schools with any educational plans that the student had during secondary education, such as an Individualized Education Plan (IEP) or Section 504 plan, although these plans may not be enough documentation for the post-secondary school. A post-secondary institution is not required to pay for any new evaluations that are needed. If a person is eligible, state vocational rehabilitation agencies may be able to assist in providing no-cost evaluations. State vocational rehabilitation agencies can be found on the internet at:

http://jan.wvu.edu/SBSES/VOCREHAB.HTM

The evaluations and documentation should also provide recommendations about necessary accommodations required for the student in the educational setting. This evaluation will assist the student in receiving appropriate services. This information should be given to the school's Disabilities Support Services. Documentation provided to the post-secondary institution cannot be more than three years old to be accepted. A school cannot deny admission to a student based on disability if he or she meets the requirements for acceptance. Unlike secondary schools, it is the student's job to inform all teachers of his or her disability and necessary accommodations.

Your Rights

Two federal laws protect students at colleges and universities. These laws include Section 504 of the 1973 Rehabilitation Act and Title II of the Americans with Disabilities Act of 1990 (P.L. 101-336).

Section 504 of the 1973 Rehabilitation Act

The Office of Civil Rights, through the U.S. Department of Education, enforces the implementation of Section 504 of the Rehabilitation Act of 1973. Section 504 "prohibits discrimination on the basis of physical or mental disability" (29 U.S.C. section 794). As stated in Section 504: "No otherwise qualified individual with a disability in the United States shall, solely by reason of his disability, be excluded from the participation in, be denied the benefits of, or be subjected to discrimination under any program or activity receiving federal financial assistance." This statement means that a post-secondary program (public or private college or university, vocational and adult education) that receives federal funds is required to provide necessary academic adjustments to limit barriers of discrimination based on a physical or mental disability and cannot deny admission based on disability if the student meets admission requirements. If a higher education institution fails to provide students with auxiliary aids that result in a "denial of program benefit," it is considered discrimination.

Americans with Disabilities Act-Title II

Title II of the Americans with Disabilities Act of 1990 (ADA) is a law protecting students from state and local government discrimination on the basis of disability. Title II is enforced in public universities and colleges and graduate and professional schools. Title II states that "a public entity shall furnish appropriate auxiliary aids and services where necessary to afford an individual with a disability an equal opportunity to participate in, and enjoy the benefits of, a service, program, or activity conducted by a public entity." In other words, the school must provide necessary auxiliary aids and services in a timely manner. While a student is being evaluated to determine if services are warranted, the student must provide his or her own auxiliary aids during that time until eligibility is established.

Obtaining Necessary Services

It is important to recognize that a person with a brain injury may require special services during school and throughout life. The student himself or herself may not recognize the difficulties. Unfortunately, there are many educational settings in which class sizes are too large and resources too limited, resulting in lack of access to necessary resources. In other cases, the services exist, but are not used effectively. In a recent study funded by the National Institute on Disability and Rehabilitation Research (NIDRR), it was found that the available services were often underutilized because of the lack of awareness, social stigma, or lack of insight into the individual's own problems or deficits. It is critical that individuals with brain injuries and their families be alert to problems with getting necessary accomodations and bringing such problems to the attention of school administrators.

Auxiliary Aids/Services

- Lighter class load (part-time studies)
- Note takers
- Method(s) used by the teacher to teach the lecture (verbal, visual, handouts, web notes)
- Reduced course loads
- Extra time for assignments
- Special seating
- Alternative test sites
- Enlarged print on tests and assignments
- Adaptive and assistive technology
- Campus transportation
- Interpreters
- Substitution of courses that aren't necessary for degree
- Electronic readers
- Assistive listening devices

Resources for Secondary Education

- College Bound Program
- Health Resource Center –www.health.gwu.edu
- Online Clearing House on Postsecondary Education for Individuals with Disabilities
- Peterson College Guide for Students with Disabilities

VOCATIONAL REHABILITATION

Traumatic brain injury is most common in the 18- to 60-year-old range, which means that many individuals were employed and will want to return to work. Therefore, returning to work is usually a primary goal for these people. However, returning to work in their previous career is not always an option because of cognitive, behavioral, emotional, vision or physical impairments that were not present prior to the brain injury. In such cases vocational rehabilitation can be a critical component to successful return to employment. Returning to work is a key goal in improving one's quality of life after a brain injury. Furthermore, it is estimated that the cost of care of people with TBI is over $60 billion per year in the United States (based on CDC report, 2000). A large portion of that cost results from loss of wages for people of employment age who can no longer work; this amount may be up to $22 billion per year in lost wages.

Americans with Disabilities Act (ADA) Title I

In the context of returning to work following a brain injury, being familiar with the basic principles of the ADA-Title I may be helpful. In summary, Title I makes it unlawful to discriminate against individuals with a disability in public and private sector employment (if the business has 15 or more employees). It is also unlawful to discriminate against an individual with a disability in state and local government services, public accommodations, transportation, or telecommunication. This act also restricts questions that can be asked about an applicant's disability before a job offer is made. It also requires that employers make reasonable accommodations for the physical or mental limitations of otherwise qualified individuals with disabilities, unless it results in undue hardship for the business. For further information on work-related rights for individuals, visit the website for the ADA at http://www.ada.gov/.

What is Vocational Rehabilitation?

Vocational rehabilitation is an approach to improve a person's ability to return to a successful vocation (e.g., return to work, job retention, etc.) following disability. In this case, the disability is the brain injury, but vocational rehabilitation is available for anyone with disability.

There are three primary types of vocational rehabilitation used for persons with brain injury: (1) program-based vocational rehabilitation, (2) supported employment, and (3) a care-coordinated approach.

The program-based approach will start with individual rehabilitation and will evaluate a person's strengths, weaknesses, interests, and pre-injury skills. The program then helps with job trials in which the individual with a brain injury may do limited tasks within a rehabilitation center or hospital-based setting. Ultimately, the program staff will help with job placement. This system provides the greatest amount of assistance and rehabilitation before starting work.

Supported employment is a system in which specialists in vocational rehabilitation accompany the person with brain injury to a new job and observe and assist them on the job to ensure that the employer is providing appropriate accommodations. The vocational specialist also assists the individual with techniques to accommodate problems that he or she may be having in completing the required job tasks. This form of rehabilitation provides the greatest amount of on-the-job rehabilitation. The vocational specialist will gradually decrease the amount of time spent at the worksite as the person demonstrates increased competency in the workplace.

The final type of vocational rehabilitation, the care-coordinated approach, is one in which the person with a brain injury is provided with his or her own care coordinator who helps with placement into the most appropriate work setting. In this type of vocational rehabilitation, the care coordinator is available to assist the individual with the brain injury, but also provides education and resources for the employer. Typically, most of the involvement of the care coordinator occurs before the person starts in the job, but the care coordinator may be re-consulted for additional assistance if needed.

At this point, it is unclear whether one of the above methods is superior to the other. Based on the literature available, it is most likely that the best style of vocational rehabilitation depends on the individual, his or her impairment, his or her learning style, the type of work, etc.

ADDITIONAL CONSIDERATIONS

The vocational and educational services in the community are available to anyone in need based on their disability. They are not dependent upon race, religion, sex, age, or ethnicity. However, there may be language (English not a first language), cultural, or socio-economic barriers (financial, transportation, etc.) that can make it more difficult for

someone with a brain injury to return successfully to work. There is
some suggestion that the initial return to work is approximately equiva-
lent when comparing Caucasians to minorities. However, there may be
a decrease in sustained employment among minorities due to some of
the factors mentioned above. It is important to remember that the educational and vocational rehabilitation services available may be utilized
at any time, not just immediately following a brain injury. So a person
who successfully returned to work may be required to adapt to a new
job responsibility in the future. This situation may be caused by a
change in job, change in the management, etc. If the person has difficulties with the new position, he or she should contact vocational services for additional assistance. It is very important that the individual, the
employer, and the vocational specialists account for the various socio-
economic, language, and cultural factors that may affect minorities out
of proportion to others who have suffered a brain injury.

Vocational rehabilitation services are available in all states. The following website provides an online listing of state vocational rehabilitation centers throughout the country:

http://www.workworld.org/wwwebhelp/state_vocational_
rehabilitation_vr_agencies.htm.

14

LIFE SKILLS AND RECREATION

HEATHER CAMPBELL

[My son] Ryan continuously challenges himself. In just the last year, he
completed three races using a hand-crank bike: the Hope and
Possibility 5K run, the Army 10 Miler, and the New York Marathon.
—Lorrie Knight-Major

If someone is asked, "What do you like to do?" most of us would not answer "work." Work is what we do to help us pay our bills and help us afford our leisure activities. Chapter 13 discusses work (vocational) rehabilitation. In this chapter, we will discuss recreation (avocational) rehabilitation. Everyone has a different idea about what "recreation" means. It can be reading, traveling, swimming, playing sports, going to a ballgame or a funny movie, watching television, attending cooking classes, biking, sailing, being with friends, working out, dancing, water skiing, painting, and much more. The list is endless.

After a traumatic brain injury, many people may feel like they cannot participate in recreational activities as they had in the past. That fact may be partially true, but there are still many opportunities for recreation, maybe some activities that were never even considered before the injury. Having a traumatic brain injury may change the way a person participates in activities, but it should not stop anyone from having fun. The changes required to participate in recreational activities may include using adaptive equipment, finding accessible facilities, having to plan ahead more, and being creative; the recreation therapists can help with these changes. Additionally, there are many community organizations that are designed specifically to provide recreational services to persons with disabilities.

This chapter shares ideas, skills, and information that can help a person who has suffered a brain injury return to a satisfying leisure life. In this chapter, the reader will learn about:

- Therapeutic recreation while in the rehabilitation hospital
- Benefits of recreational activities
- Options for recreational activities
- Planning for recreational activities
- Where to look for recreation opportunities

THERAPEUTIC RECREATION WHILE IN AN INPATIENT SETTING

Leisure time is free time during which one can do what he or she wants to do. Recreation is what is done during the leisure time. It is an individual's decision how to use his leisure time. He or she can spend it alone, with family, friends, or others who have similar interests.

While in the rehabilitation hospital, patients are introduced to recreational activities by a recreational therapist (RT). Recreation therapy is the implementation of recreational activities as an intervention with the purpose of maintaining or improving health, functional ability, active leisure lifestyle, and quality of life for the patient. Therapeutic recreation is provided by professionals who are trained and certified, registered, or licensed to provide this service. Therapeutic recreation is used to help reach the primary goal of rehabilitation, which is using skills and interests that were present prior to the injury to regain independent functioning while adjusting to an altered lifestyle. The RT will work with a person after an injury to return to the leisure and community activities he or she did prior to the injury. The person with brain injury will also have the opportunity to try new leisure activities, adapt activities that he or she enjoyed before the injury, and learn where to participate in activities in the local area.

Recreation might be the last thing on a person's mind during a hospital stay. However, by participating in the activities offered, he or she will be working on therapy goals while having fun. In addition, as a part of recreational therapy, he or she may also have the opportunity to take part in activities in the local community through a community skills outing. These activities might include going to the mall, going bowling, going to a museum, or eating out. One may be nervous at first, but most people return from these community outings more relaxed and feeling more prepared to return home. Experiencing the community for the first time since the accident is easier with the therapists.

THE IMPORTANCE OF RETURNING TO LEISURE ACTIVITIES

Participation in recreational and leisure activities offers many advantages that enhance one's physical, cognitive, social, and emotional state, all of which improve one's overall quality of life. For example, participation in leisure activities gives a person the chance to learn new skills, meet or socialize with other people, and improve his physical health. Participation in recreational activities is also vital to one's overall well-being. Research suggests that participation in exercise activities can help prevent secondary medical conditions such as cardiovascular disease, urinary tract infections, development of high blood pressure, depression, deconditioning (getting out of shape), and obesity. It also provides mental health benefits. It can also decrease social isolation, strengthen community living skills, and help promote advocacy for those people living with a TBI. Gaining these benefits from leisure activities is even more important for those with brain injury who may be limited in the pursuit of daily occupation or education. Leisure activities then become the source for self-fulfillment and reinforcement.

Experts often emphasize the importance of physical activity for good health, but going to the gym, lifting weights, or playing sports is not everyone's idea of fun. One can get many of the same benefits by participating in less strenuous recreational activities that may be of more interest to some people. The Surgeon General has reported that significant health benefits can be obtained with a moderate amount of daily physical activity. All it takes is 30 minutes a day to help prevent disease. Actually, any increase in physical activity can help a person feel better. Think about shopping, traveling, bowling, gardening, or walking the dog. All of these activities get you moving and at the same time increase your overall conditioning.

ACTIVITIES FOR DISABLED PERSONS

Many people who have suffered a brain injury find that they have a less active lifestyle after the injury than they did before. They find themselves more sedentary which leads to the body becoming deconditioned. In turn, this change in physical well-being will lead to increased dependence on others for routine daily activities. People with brain injuries have an increased risk of developing poor health habits, particularly regarding exercise and physical activities.

The complications of inactivity, which affect both body and mind, can by prevented by developing a regular exercise program. The National Center for Physical Activity and Disability (NCPAD) states that the best exercise program for individuals with brain injury includes stretching, strength training, and cardiovascular training. It is important to start with a stretching program because most people with brain injury have been sedentary for long periods of time. Once comfortable with the stretching, one can move on to a strength training program in which he or she can do something as simple as using therapeutic bands at home to work all muscle groups. Reaching the cardiovascular part of the program does not mean one has to go out and run. Other ways to get cardiovascular training include walking, riding a stationary recumbent bike, water aerobics, gardening, and shopping. NCPAD recommends a proper medical referral and health evaluation screening prior to implementing any fitness regimen. Any current health or physical limitation should be properly managed under the supervision of a medical professional.

OUTDOOR ACTIVITIES: HEAD FOR THE GREAT OUTDOORS

Sailing, canoeing, hiking, camping, visiting the beach, gardening, and other outdoor activities are all still possible after a brain injury. Many national and local community organizations provide information about these activities and offer opportunities to try the adaptive equipment needed to participate in such activities. These organizations are also a way to meet other people with similar interests in your area.

For example, there are organizations that offer year-round activities in snow skiing, water skiing, sailing, kayaking, white water rafting and handcycling, among others. For a small fee these groups will provide instruction and the adaptive equipment necessary to participate. Through such organizations, you can participate in all these activities with family and friends.

Your recreation therapist can provide many ideas and information about how to get involved. The internet is also a great source for locating such organizations.

ACCESS IS GETTING BETTER

Since the Americans with Disabilities Act (ADA) became a law in 1990, opportunities for leisure activities for people with disabilities have grown exponentially. For example:

- Most performing arts theaters and concert venues provide accessible wheelchair seating. Some even have specially priced tickets for people with disabilities.
- Most stadiums and sports arenas have an accessibility office that can assist with getting accessible seating to watch a favorite team. Anyone can call their office ahead of time, or take a ticket for regular seating to the office once he arrives to the game to have it exchanged for an accessible seat.
- Many malls now offer walking programs that take place early in the morning and provide a safe, level, air-conditioned walking environment. It is a great way to build endurance and strength. It is also a great opportunity for meeting new people.
- Movie theaters now have accessible seats in the front, middle, and back. Theaters have removed three or more seats, so someone with disabilities can sit in a wheelchair next to the person with whom he or she came.

As you can see, opportunities for recreation really are endless. The key is to get moving. People with a brain injury should think of all the things they enjoy doing and all the things they always wanted to do. Now, make a plan.

MAKE A PLAN

Even if a person who has had a brain injury was not particularly recreation-oriented in the past, now is a great opportunity to get started. This section offers the tools to start making a recreation plan that is realistic, but still suits the personal needs and interests of the person with a brain injury. There are three steps to get the person thinking about recreational activities, where one can get them, and how one is going to do them! The steps are:

Step 1: Choose an activity.
Step 2: Find a place where it can be done.
Step 3: Identify potential barriers and find solutions.

Step 1: Choose an Activity

As planning begins, get back to basics. The person planning the recreation should think about the reasons he or she wants to participate in recreational activities. Is it to find new friends who share similar interests? Is it to find new ways to relax or feel a sense of achievement? Is it just to enjoy nature? Or, is it to find others recovering from and living with a brain injury? Remember that sometimes after an injury, a person's needs may be different from what they were before the injury. The reasons for participating in certain activities may be different now.

Before choosing an activity for participation, one should first identify which goals he or she wants to achieve with the activity. Is it to gain strength? Gain endurance? Or just have some fun? Next, he or she should identify his or her strengths and limitations in order to modify the chosen activity as needed for successful participation. Use the checklist in Table 14.1 below to assess the reasons you want to participate in recreational activities.

After identifying the reasons for participating in recreational activities, use Table 14.2 for potential opportunities. This table is not meant to be comprehensive, but rather to give some ideas of appropriate activities to meet the desired goals. Remember to try any activity that sounds fun. It is important to find activities that can be enjoyed with family and friends.

After choosing an activity, break down the components of the activity. By breaking the activity into smaller pieces, it is easier to plan for par-

Table 14.1. Reasons to participate in recreational activities.

THE TOP REASONS TO PARTICIPATE IN RECREATIONAL ACITIVITIES ARE TO:
• Be more physically active • Be around people and socialize • Reduce stress and relax • Feel a sense of achievement • Enjoy nature

Table 14.2. A list of activities based on personal goals.

Personal goal desired to achieve with activity:	Activities to consider:
Be more physically active	• Join a gym/exercise class • Work out with an exercise video • Kayak, canoe, or sail • Hike • Ride a recumbent bike
Be around people and socialize	• Join a club • Take a class (such as a computer, painting, or crafts) • Attend a worship service • Be a volunteer
Reduce stress and relax	• Take a water exercise class • Garden • See a movie or a play • Paint
Feel a sense of achievement	• Be a volunteer • Take a class • Complete a project
Enjoy nature	• Hike • Travel • Canoe, sail, or kayak • Camp
Be adventurous	• Travel to exotic places • Take a hot air balloon ride • Ski

ticipation. Examples of things you want to ask yourself include: What skills does it take to do the activity? Can the person with a disability do the activity himself or does it involve other people? Can he or she find people in the community who can help to learn the activity?

Step 2: Find Places Where You Can Do It

After a person has identified a recreational activity he or she wants to do, he or she will need to figure out where appropriate facilities are available. Below is a list of some of the many places in your community that may offer recreation activities:

- Community centers
- City or county recreation departments (Contact the therapeutic recreation office for specific information on adapted recreation and accessible pools and facilities.)
- YMCAs and YWCAs
- Universities and community colleges
- Fitness clubs
- Shopping malls (walking programs)
- Libraries (offer free Internet access, book groups, and lectures)
- Craft stores (offer classes)
- Theaters
- Museums
- Volunteer service organizations
- Hospitals (may offer workshops and fitness centers)
- Golf courses (many have accessible carts)
- Tennis clubs
- Garden clubs
- Horseback riding stables
- Travel groups

To find out more information about other activities in your area:

- Get on the mailing lists of adapted sports organizations and local parks and recreation departments. These newsletters may spark an interest in something new.

- Look in the Yellow Pages to find places that offer recreational activities.
- Read your local newspaper, including activity listings.
- Ask friends or other people with disabilities where they go for recreational activities.
- Talk with recreation therapists at the rehabilitation hospital.
- For any organization that has activities of interest, contact the national organization to locate chapters in the local area.
- Search in the internet (using the activity name and the city/community name as search terms).

Questions to ask when contacting places that offer recreational activities in the community include:

- Where are you located?
- What recreational activities do you offer?
- Are your facilities and programs accessible to people in wheelchairs?
- What accommodations do you offer for people with disabilities?
- Do you have any adaptive equipment that I can use?
- Is the program open to everyone or is it only for persons with disabilities?
- How much does it cost?
- What are the times and dates of programs?
- How do I register?
- Can I be added to your mailing list?

Some of the factors that will determine which locations are best suited for the needs of an individual will be determined in step 3 below.

Step 3: Identify Barriers and Find Solutions

Have you ever heard yourself think or say "I can't because….!" Almost everyone has said this at one time or another. Many factors can prevent someone with a disability from continuing an activity or taking up a new activity, whether it's playing a sport with friends, working out regularly at the gym, going dancing, or doing a craft. Anyone can come up with a physical, psychological, or other reason not to do something, but sometimes it is just a matter of finding a workable solution to motivate a person to get involved. It is important to identify the barriers up front and then find solutions to break down the barriers. With some thought and creativity, one can turn "I can't!" into "I can!"

Step 3 in the planning process consists of taking steps to get involved in the recreational activity or activities the person with the injury has chosen. The first part of this step is to identify those barriers that could prevent someone from doing the activity and looking for solutions that will help to get him or her involved. Common barriers to participation in recreational activities include lack of money, transportation problems, lack of affordable adaptive equipment, and having no one with whom he or she can enjoy the activity. Below are some possible solutions to help break down these barriers and get started.

I Don't Have Enough Money . . .

Not having enough extra money to participate in an activity is a factor for many people. Equipment costs and admission fees can really add up. Search for free or low-cost activities in the local community. Ideas for finding inexpensive activities include:

- Check the local newspaper for notices about free or low-cost events, or for discount coupons.
- Contact theaters in the area to find out about special discounts that they may offer. Remember to ask about wheelchair accessibility, if necessary.
- Check with recreational organizations to find out if they will wave membership fees or offer some sort of scholarship program.
- Ask organizations about attending events free for volunteering.
- Ask about tuition assistance for classes.

I Can't Get There . . .

Handicapped accessibility on public transportation has greatly improved over the past few years. In major metropolitan areas, subways and buses are accessible for people in wheelchairs. Buses are equipped with ramps and lockdowns for wheelchairs. Subway trains are accessible with elevators available to get to and from the train. Contact your local public transportation office and inquire about travel training in your area. In Washington, D.C., the Washington Metropolitan Area Transit Authority offers travel training. Many cities will offer such training. Problems still exist when their elevators or ramps break down, but they will still provide an alternative route for people with disabilities. Many people successfully use public transportation on a regular basis.

As required by the ADA, cities also offer paratransit services. These low-cost services provide curb-to-curb or door-to-door transportation for individuals with disabilities who qualify. Check with the local county or city government for information about paratransit services in the area. When using paratransit services, be sure to schedule well in advance and allow ample time to be picked up in order to arrive at the destination on time. As a person with a disability becomes more independent with wheelchair skills, using a public bus or subway may be a better option because it allows one to set his or her own schedule, and it is less expensive. Also, once the person with a brain injury has a MetroAccess ID card, this individual and one other person can ride the public bus or subway for free.

Also check with local taxi services. Many taxi companies offer accessible services. Additionally, if one is planning to attend a sports clinic or support group meeting, check with the leaders of the event to see if carpooling is a possibility.

I Don't Have the Right Equipment . . .

Getting access to adaptive equipment and finding affordable equipment to buy can sometimes be challenging. Check with local sports and recreation organizations for persons with disabilities to see if they have any ideas about where to borrow or buy equipment. Many have adaptive equipment that they loan to members participating in events. If one attends an introductory clinic or class for a sport or other activity of interest, he or she can ask the instructors about where to buy good, used equipment.

Fortunately, it is not necessary to reinvent the wheel when it comes to adapting recreational activities to meet the needs of people with brain injury. Many people have already done this and "know the ropes." Contact a recreation therapist in the local area for help with finding out more about adaptive activities. National and local organizations also can provide information and answer many questions related to these activities. For example, the National Center for Physical Activity and Disability (http://www.ncpad.org) has compiled information about a variety of recreational activities and sports. A virtually unlimited number of resources are available online which can be accessed through the internet.

To participate in some activities, one may need adaptive equipment, such as a playing card holder, an adapted fishing rod, a handle grip for bowling, a sit ski, adapted computer equipment or longer adapted gardening tools. To assist with obtaining the appropriate equipment, one can discuss his or her needs with the recreation therapists or rehabilitation engineers at a rehabilitation hospital to find low-cost ways to adapt equipment. Special organizations provide qualified instructions in activities. By participating in their events one can test equipment to identify what works best without having to purchase the items first.

I Don't Have Anyone to Do It With . . .

This one is relatively easy! The person with a brain injury can join an organization or club where one meets other people with similar interests. He or she could take a class and have fun learning a new skill with other novices. Another option would be to join a TBI support group where one can meet and learn from others with TBI. Often support groups sponsor get-together social events as well. In addition, he or she might volunteer with an organization to meet people with similar enthusiasm for a certain activity. The more a person with a brain injury gets out and participates in the community, the more people he or she will meet.

PUTTING IT ALL TOGETHER

Now that the brain injury survivor has thought through the types of activities that interests him or her, gathered information about where to do the activities, what adaptations are needed, and determined how barriers can be overcome, it is time to act on the plan.

Become an Advocate

As one returns to his or her community, an individual may find that some places he or she would have liked to have gone are not accessible. If this happens, one should not give up. Even if he or she has never done so before, he or she should become an advocate. A person who has survived a brain injury is his or her own best advocate. If one had a previous relationship with a place to which he or she would like to return, he or she should talk with the owner or management. Explain what is preventing a disabled person from coming to the place of business. The staff may be unaware that a problem exists until someone speaks up. Often, they will consider making reasonable changes so that people with brain injuries and other disabilities can use their facilities.

Now Go Do It!

Although school, work, and other obligations are very important, it is still important to make relaxation and social enjoyment a priority in one's life. Remember how important it is, both mentally and physically, for someone to remain active after a brain injury. No one really wants to stay home and stare at the four walls. In the beginning, everything may seem to be harder, take longer, and be exhausting, but as with everything else accomplished through rehabilitation, participation in recreational activities also will become easier. As the needed skills are acquired and endurance improves, a person with a brain injury can have a full, rewarding lifestyle. Take small steps: go to a movie, a restaurant, to a ball game or a friend's house. Just take the time to carefully plan the activities in advance to ensure success.

What Can I Do?

As one makes choices about physical and recreational activities be sure to:

- Find activities the person enjoys doing. If one is having fun, he or she will be more likely to stick with it and do it more often.
- Be creative. Where there is a will, there is a way. If one really likes to do something, he or she should find a new way to do it. Get ideas

from therapists and others with similar disabilities and similar interests.

- Plan ahead. Check on accessibility and plan transportation in advance.
- Be flexible. Do not give up just because the transportation is late. Have a "Plan B."
- Find someone to accompany the individual with the brain injury. Many activities are more fun with family and friends.
- Set goals. Set reasonable goals regarding how much one can accomplish in a day. When these goals have been met, set new ones.
- Get connected. Sign up for mailing lists for support groups, special organizations, and clubs. If their newsletters come to the home, sooner or later something will spark his or her interest.
- Know the individual. Be aware of specific needs and limits.
- Strive for balance. Try to balance rest and recreation. Rest will be important during recovery, but too much will set him or her back. Ask the therapists for ideas, activities and exercises within his or her limits. Do not reach for the remote!
- Let others know what is needed. The person with a brain injury is his best spokesperson. Let friends and family know when help is needed and when it is not.
- Challenge. Use extra time to try a new activity, learn a new language, or see a new place.

KEY POINTS

- Physical and recreational activities offer many benefits, including the chance to learn new skills, relax, meet and socialize with others, and improve or maintain your physical and mental health.
- Leisure activities include everything from strength training and outdoor sports to shopping and walking the dog.
- Good planning can help one become more active and enjoy his leisure time more. To make a plan, learn about activities that seem enjoyable, find places or organizations that can help one get involved, and be creative in overcoming barriers that may prevent someone from getting started.

—15—
PATIENT RESOURCES

KIMBERLY LOCKETT

*I know I can't change the world, but I felt certain I could and would
do all I could to change my son's world.* —Maryann Griswold

It is in the period shortly after a brain
injury when survivors and their families are under the most stress. The
stresses can vary from emotional, psychological, or physical stressors to
financial ones. Often, because of the brain injury, one of the bread-win-
ning members of the family is unable to work and earn a salary. At other
times, a young person with a brain injury is left to take care of his or her
financial needs and affairs by himself or herself. This time is critical to
find out about some of the community resources that can be used to
meet the needs of the individual with a brain injury. This chapter provides much information about accessing such services; however, it is not
meant to be all-inclusive. This chapter will cover resources that are
available to assist persons with disability throughout the United States.
Also, many local and regional services are not covered in this chapter.
One can find additional resources on the internet and the library, or by
asking the social workers or case managers.

HEALTHCARE PLANS

There are several different types of health insurance. Some insurance
companies may offer different plans so it is important to know not only
what insurance company provides coverage for the person with the
brain injury, but also what different plan options are available. Types of
health insurance include fee-for-service or managed care. Managed
care plans are further divided into Health Maintenance Organizations
(HMOs), Point-of-Service (POS) options, and Preferred Provider

Organizations (PPOs). In addition to the plan types mentioned here, different types of payers are discussed below.

Private Insurance

Health insurance is available through a variety of private entities, including not-for-profit organizations, for-profit organizations, and for-profit companies. These organizations offer a wide range of fee-for-services and managed-care plans, including group plans (such as those provided through employers and unions) and individual plans. Each insurer's plans differ from other insurers.

In addition to setting limits on individual covered benefits, many private fee-for-service and managed-care plans set limits, called "caps" on the dollar amount they will pay each year or over a person's lifetime. On the other hand, most private health insurance policies have catastrophic limits of coverage. These limits place a ceiling on the out-of-pocket expenses that you must pay for medical services and prescription drugs. The limits include any premiums, deductibles, and co-payments that you have contributed toward your care. Fee-for-service plans generally set higher catastrophic limits of coverage than those set by managed-care plans.

Most private health-insurance plans cover skilled nursing care received in a nursing home as long as it is prescribed following a hospital stay. However, custodial care received in a nursing home, long-term care facility, or at home generally is not covered by private health insurance plans. Custodial care is care provided mainly to help people take care of their daily needs (eating, bathing, and dressing) and does not cover required treatment or services from specially training professionals, such as doctors, therapists, or nurses.

Medicare

Medicare was created under the Social Security Act of 1965 as a national health insurance program aimed at ensuring basic health care for people aged 65 or older and those disabled for at least two years. Medicare is funded entirely by the federal government. As is the case with private insurance, insured people pay deductibles and co-payments for most types of services. Medicare has two main parts. As long as you have both Part A and Part B, items covered by either part remain covered whether you have the original Medicare plan, or you belong to a Medicare Advantage Plan (like an HMO or PPO).

Medicare Part A

Part A (hospital insurance) helps pay for care in hospitals as an inpatient, critical access hospitals (small facilities that give limited outpatient and inpatient services to people in rural areas), skilled nursing facilities (not custodial or long-term care), hospice care, and some home health care. If you are not sure if the patient has Part A, look on the red, white, and blue Medicare card. If he or she has this coverage, "HOSPITAL (PART A)" is printed on the card.

Most people get Part A automatically when they turn age 65. They do not have to pay a monthly payment called a premium for Part A because they or a spouse paid Medicare taxes while they were working. If one does not automatically get premium-free Part A, he or she may be able to buy it. No cost Part A Medicare is only available to people who worked and paid enough in Medicare taxes while they were employed. Another reason that one may not have premium-free Part A after the age of 65 is if he or she returned to work. If he or she has limited income and resources, the state may help him or her pay for Part A and/or Part B.

Medicare Part B

Medicare Part B (medical insurance) helps pay for doctors' services, outpatient care, and other medical services that Part A does not cover. Part B helps pay for these covered medical services and items when they are medically necessary. Part B also covers some preventive services.

The Part B premiums vary by income and whether a person files taxes as an individual or a couple. In some cases this amount may be higher if one did not choose Part B when he or she first became eligible. The cost of Part B may go up 10% for each full 12-month period that he or she could have had Part B but did not sign up for it, except in special cases. You may have to pay this penalty as long as you have Part B.

Enrolling in Part B is the individual's choice. A person can sign up for Part B from three months before he or she turns 65 to three months after that date. To sign up, call the Social Security Administration at 1-800-772-1213 or visit or call the local Social Security office.

Medigap Supplement Insurance

Original Medicare does not cover deductibles, doctor and hospital co-insurance or co-payment, or emergency care outside the country. However, most "Medigap" plans do. When shopping for such a plan, make sure it is clearly identified as "Medicare Supplement Insurance." This supplemental coverage is available through private insurance companies and some private organizations, including the AMA (American Medical Association) and AARP (formerly the American Association for Retired Persons). When one signs up for Medicare Part B, he or she automatically begins a six-month Medigap open enrollment period. Once that period begins, it cannot be changed or restarted. If he or she has enrolled in a Medicare Advantage plan, it is illegal for anyone to sell him a Medigap policy.

There are 10 different types of Medigap plans, labeled A-J. Plan A offers the fewest benefits and is usually the least expensive; Plan J offers the most benefits and is usually the most expensive. All of the plans must include the following basic benefits: hospital coinsurance coverage; 365 days of full hospital coverage over and above the patient's lifetime coverage as a Medicare enrollee to be used after he or she uses all Medicare hospital benefits; 20 percent of the cost of one's medical care that Medicare does not pick up after the $110 deductible is paid; and the first three pints of blood you need each year. Depending on which Medigap plan he or she has, a person can get extra coverage for hospital deductibles; skilled nursing facility coinsurance; emergency care outside the United States; costs associated with recovering at home; Part B excess charges; preventive care; and limited prescription drug coverage.

Medicare Part D

Medicare Part D is a prescription drug plan offered by insurance companies and other private companies approved by Medicare. With such a plan, a beneficiary still must pay a co-payment, coinsurance, and/or deductible. If he or she has limited income and resources, he or she may be able to receive help to pay for the Medicare drug plan costs. For general Medicare information and information about health plans, contact 1-800-MEDICARE (1-800-633-4227) 24 hours a day, 7 days a week for assistance.

Medicaid

Medicaid is a welfare health care program that is administered by each state with cofunding provided by the federal government. There are three types of Medicaid: (1) Community Based, (2) Custodial Long-Term Care, and (3) Waiver Programs.

Medicaid does not pay money directly to the patient; instead, it sends payments directly to his or her healthcare providers. Depending on the state's Medicaid rules, one may also be required to pay a small part of the cost (co-payment) for certain medical services. Medicaid can be used as a secondary insurance as well. Eligibility varies from state to state, but is always based on particular medical, financial, and age criteria. To qualify for Medicaid, the recipient must be disabled and have a limited amount in countable resources. Some variations by state in resource limitations apply, but individuals who do not meet these criteria can be denied Medicaid. To apply, he or she will need to complete an application form and bring the following documentation to the local Medicaid office:

- Proof of income (for example, pay stubs or proof of retirement income, disability income, or Worker's Compensation)
- Proof of your assets (for example, banking and checking account statements)
- Proof of residence (for example, utility or telephone bill, lease, rent receipt, or driver's license)
- Proof of your Social Security number (for example, Social Security card or other official documents with your Social Security number on it)
- Medicare card, if applicable
- All medical bills received

Medicaid Home and Community Based Services (HCBS) Waiver

The Medicaid HCBS Waiver program allows state Medicaid agencies to request waivers under Section 1915(c) of the Social Security Act. This program offers community-based services as an alternative to institutional care provided in a nursing facility, ICF/MR (intermediate care facility for those developmentally delayed), or a hospital. These waiver programs permit an individual who meets the requirements for admission to an institutional setting to receive appropriate services and support in his or her home or a community-based setting and maintain both independence and ties to family and friends. To be a waiver participant, an individual must be medically qualified, certified for the waiver's institutional level of care, and choose to enroll in the waiver as an alternative to institutionalization. Financially, one must meet eligibility based on income and assets. The age of the individual at the time of the brain injury, as well as any other diagnosis a person may have, is also significant and will determine which waiver a person would be eligible for. The cost to Medicaid must be no more in the community under the waiver than in an institution. Each HCBS waiver may include different services targeted to the population being served and may include services, such as case management, homemaker services, home health aide services, personal care, adult day health care, habilitation, vocational rehabilitation and respite care, or other services defined by the state and authorized by CMS (the Centers for Medicare and Medicaid Services). The services may be provided by a number of different providers and vary in scope and intensity depending on the needs of the beneficiary. The populations served under HCBS waivers vary by state.

Workers' Compensation

Under Workers' Compensation law, an employee is eligible for compensation for injuries or diseases caused by work. For an injury to be covered, it must have occurred while working; it must be caused by a work activity; and it must have occurred suddenly and accidentally. For a disease to be covered, it needs to be caused by work activity, but it does not have to be caused by a specific accident. Employees receive different benefits depending on the severity and permanency of the impairment. These benefits can include medical care and hospitalization, wage replacement, vocational rehabilitation, and death benefits. To receive benefits, employees must inform their employer and file a claim as soon as possible. The employee or his or her representative should contact the local Workers' Compensation Commission for detailed information. The contact information can be found on the internet, in a local telephone directory, or by calling information (411).

TRICARE

TRICARE is the health plan for the U.S. Military. TRICARE provides services throughout the military system as well as insurance coverage for eligible members to receive services in the civilian sector. To be eligible for TRICARE, you must be active duty military, retired (length of service) military, certain medically retired service members, or dependents (family members) of military members

Veterans Affairs (VA)

The U.S. Department of Veterans Affairs is responsible for the medical and rehabilitative care of millions of U.S. veterans. The majority of VA services are provided directly through the VA system; however, they do outsource to civilian providers if the services are not available within the VA system. Dependents of veterans are not eligible for veterans health services. The VA system has a very long history of providing rehabilitation services. The VA currently has four Polytrauma Medical Centers that specialize in rehabilitation of the veterans with traumatic brain injury. These centers are located in Richmond, Virginia; Tampa, Forida; Minneapolis, Minnesota; and Palo Alto, California. Seventeen additional Polytrauma Network Sites are located throughout the United States.

ALTERNATIVE FINANCIAL RESOURCES

Despite having insurance, sometimes not all services are covered. After a serious medical event, such as a brain injury, financial drain may be an issue that affects the family's ability to pay for many services, not just medical care. The Department of Social Services in the local areas provides a variety of services and programs to eligible residents. Programs such as Temporary Assistance for Needy Families (TANF), food stamps, energy assistance, Medicaid, and others are managed and implemented by each state. To apply for assistance, contact the local department of social services in person or visit online. Some agencies require an interview by an eligibility worker, depending on the type of assistance you are requesting. If the person with the brain injury is not able to be interviewed, a family member can be interviewed to provide the necessary information. Some of the types of services that are available include:

- Basic Needs: programs that provide food, diapers, and clothing
- Day Care Services: programs to assist with child care or adult day care
- State Programs: food stamps, health services (Medicaid and Medicare), legal help in obtaining child support, unemployment benefits, etc.
- Energy Assistance: assistance with home energy needs
- Financial Assistance: programs that can help with rent, utilities, credit card balances, and other expenses in an emergency; help with budgeting, credit counseling, and debt management
- Support Services: assistance for dealing with the problems of life, including companionship, family support, addictions, and mental health

SOCIAL SECURITY

The Social Security Administration is responsible for two major programs that provide benefits based on disability: Social Security Disability Insurance (SSDI), which is based on prior work under Social Security, and Supplemental Security Income (SSI). Under SSI, payments are made on the basis of financial need.

Social Security Disability Insurance (SSDI) is financed with Social Security taxes paid by workers, employers, and self-employed persons. To be eligible for a SSDI, the worker must have earned sufficient credits based on taxable work. Disability benefits are payable to blind or disabled workers, widow(er)s, children of disabled worker, or adults disabled since childhood. The amount of the monthly disability benefit is based on the individual's lifetime average earnings covered by Social Security.

Supplemental Security Income (SSI) is a program financed through general revenues. SSI disability benefits are payable to adults or children who are disabled or blind and who meet specific income and resources requirements. Some income and assets are not counted (such as a person's home). The monthly payment varies up to the maximum federal benefit rate, which may be supplemented by the state or decreased by countable income and resources.

If one has been approved for SSDI or SSI, he or she will receive a monthly benefit amount determined by the Social Security Office. In most cases, he or she will also receive a certain amount in past due benefits based on how long it has taken the case to be resolved and when it was determined the disability actually began. This payment is received as a lump sum and, depending on its size, may be broken into installments. (SSI back payments may be paid in installments, while social security disability back payments are paid in a single lump sum.)

Disability recipients also receive certain medical benefits. Recipients whose benefits derive from SSI may receive Medicaid (depending on the state in which they live). Those whose benefits derive from the SSDI will receive Medicare. However, Medicare benefits do not become available until 2 years after gaining eligibility for social security disability benefits. This ruling does not mean that Medicare benefits become available 2 years after payments have started, but, rather 2 years after the estimated onset of disability date (based on review of medical evidence) plus a 5-month waiting period.

Ten Tips When Applying for Social Security

The application process for Social Security Disability or Social Security Income can be very challenging. The following section will provide useful information to help get through the application process.

Tip 1

The Social Security representative may not know the specifics about a person's case or may just make a human error. Therefore, when in doubt, do not hesitate to ask the same question again, or refer the same question to a different worker at the social security office or to the individual providing representation for the SSD or SSI claim.

Tip 2

Get copies of the medical records and supply these along with the SSD or SSI disability application. Frequently examiners will make decisions on claims without all of the medical evidence because he or she was unsuccessful in getting the records from a particular doctor's office, clinic, or hospital. Individuals should get records directly from the doctor or hospital and submit them with the application or appeal. Alternately, an attorney or non-attorney representative can accomplish this task. He or she should ensure that all of their records are evaluated, and that the social security disability case will not sit around for months longer than necessary.

Tip 3

Respond to all letters and notices regarding the disability case promptly.

Tip 4

If denied for SSDI or SSI, file an appeal. Some people who are denied on an initial claim for social security disability or SSI benefits go down to their local Social Security Office and complete a new application. This is a mistake. Do not do this. Filling out another disability application will only mean that the case will be denied again. By doing so, the applicant will give up his or her right to an appeal. In the event that one is denied the initial claim, the applicant should file a Request for Reconsideration. This is the first step in the Social Security Administration's appeal process. The reconsideration may also be denied, but if it is, he or she will have the right to request a Social Security Disability hearing before an administrative law judge. This hearing is where he or she will have the best chance of winning a SSD or SSI case.

Tip 5

Call Disability Determination Services (DDS) for updates on the SSD or SSI claim, not the local Social Security Office. In most cases, it is pointless to contact Social Security for status updates on a SSDI or SSI claim because that office simply will not know the answers to the questions. The DDS Examiner (the individual who actually works on the claim for disability benefits) can be called for accurate status updates. In any state, the number for DDS can always be obtained from its local Social Security Office.

Tip 6

If one has dire financial problems and a disability case, let the local Social Security office know. For the most part, a disability claimant's financial situation will have no bearing on the pace at which a SSDI or SSI disability case is processed. However, if a disability claimant is waiting for a hearing to be scheduled with an administrative law judge, the hearing can sometimes be expedited by submitting what is known as a "dire need" letter. In a dire need letter, point out why waiting the normal amount of time for a hearing (unfortunately, normal can sometimes be a year or longer) might have dire financial consequences. In most cases, this dire need means something on the order of a home foreclosure, an eviction from an apartment, or not being able to obtain prescriptions that are desperately needed. Keep in mind that the letters that get the most attention and are the most effective are the ones that have the most detail and with documentation attached. Examples of such documentation include copies of past due notices, eviction threats, foreclosure proceedings, and the like. Always keep a copy of the dire need letter you submit. After the letter is submitted, be sure to follow up on it a couple weeks later to make sure it has been received.

Tip 7

If the applicant has representation on a Social Security Disability or SSI disability case, always keep the attorney or non-attorney representative updated on what is happening with the situation, medically or otherwise.

Tip 8

If the disabled person has child support obligations that he or she cannot fulfill, ask the representative to submit a letter on his or her behalf to a child support enforcement case worker or a judge. In most instances, while a disability case is pending, such statements can keep a claimant's nonsupport status from resulting in incarceration or other penalties.

Tip 9

Get the applicant's doctor to write a supporting statement for his SSD or SSI case. The disability claims are won and lost on the basis of a claimant's medical records, including treatment notes, lab reports, x-rays, MRI studies, and statements from the doctor. If the doctor is willing to provide a statement in support of the social security disability claim, the doctor must state why the claimant is unable to work. Typically, the social security administration is looking for a doctor's evaluation of how well an SSD or SSI disability claimant can do physical work, such as sitting, standing, bending, walking, stooping, reaching overhead, lifting as well as general strength, grip strength, and range of motion.

Unfortunately, many doctors will balk at having to write this type of detailed statement, even though it is exactly what the social security administration is looking for. Nevertheless, claimants who are seriously interested in winning their SSDI and SSI claims should strive to obtain this type of statement from their doctor.

Tip 10

Make sure the doctor really does support the SSD or SSI disability case. If the doctor feels that the claimant is actually able to return to some type of employment, they are required by law to document this belief and the claimant will lose his or her case.

Additional Information: To get more information or to apply for Social Security Disability Insurance (SSDI) or Supplemental Security Income (SSI) the person with the disability or his or her representative should contact the Social Security Administration at (800) 772-1213 or www.ssa.gov. One may also contact the local Social Security office.

PRESCRIPTION DRUG ASSISTANCE

Most states have prescription drug programs to help people obtain the necessary medications for their condition. The medications available (the formulary) varies from state to state and program to program. The individual's doctor may need to change some of the recommended medications to a similar one on the program's formulary.

If the person does not qualify for government support through a pharmacy assistance program, many pharmaceutical companies have programs to assist in providing medications that they sell. One should check directly with the company for details. Information is usually available on their websites. Some large regional or national chain pharmacies now offer low price prescriptions for a selection of generic medications. These include, but are not limited to, Target, Wal-Mart, and Safeway. If an individual needs to rely on these services to obtain medication, the doctor should be notifired so he or she can prescribe medications that are on that specific plan.

VICTIM ASSISTANCE, COMPENSATION, AND STATE PROGRAMS

The person who suffered a traumatic brain injury may have been a victim of a crime and, therefore, may be eligible for certain benefits or compensation as a result. The Crime Victims Compensation Program (CVCP) assists victims and their families with the financial burden of a violent crime. The CVCP pays bills that are not covered by collateral sources such as private health, automobile or life insurance, medical aid programs, and Social Security Income or Disability. The CVCP may provide financial assistance for the following expenses:

- Crime-related medical and mental-health counseling bills
- Funeral and burial costs
- Wage support or services lost as a direct result of the crime
- Crime scene cleaning costs

- Replacement costs for clothing held as evidence
- Temporary emergency housing for domestic violence victims

If someone sustained a brain injury as a result of a crime he or she may qualify for compensation. For more information, contact the crime victim program in his or her state of residence.

GOING HOME AFTER A BRAIN INJURY

Many people who have suffered a moderate to severe brain injury may require 24 hour supervision or assistance. For some, they may only need it for a few days or weeks; others may need it for months, years, or permanently. Of course, this kind of care creates a problem for families in which the potential caretakers must work to support the household. This situation may be even more of a problem if the injured person was one of the breadwinners for the family. Therefore, it is important to find out about different resources that can provide the necessary services either within the home or through day program services. Sometimes the needs are such that it is not feasible to live at home. Other residential options are discussed below.

Home Care

After being discharged from the hospital and sometimes for a long time, people with brain injury may need help at home. Some private agencies provide in-home nursing services. Home Health Agencies (HHA) provide care in the home for individuals who are homebound because of illness or disability. Some agencies may have staff familiar with the needs of people with brain injuries, while others may not. Call the agency for more information. Most Home Health Agencies provide Personal Assistance Services for a fee or, if eligible, a person may receive these services under Medicaid or a Medicaid Waiver program.

Behavioral Home Health Services are mental health services provided in the home when an individual is homebound because of physical, medical, or psychiatric limitations. Each agency offers slightly different services that are provided under the direction/prescription of a physician.

Day Care

Adult day care programs offer a variety of services, which may include physical and occupational therapies, crafts, day trips, and other social and recreational activities. Some programs, however, do not necessarily have staff who are knowledgeable about brain injury. It is important to remember that not all programs include therapy in their daily programming. It is also important to visit the program and talk with administrators and staff about their ability to care for the needs of the person with a brain injury.

Residential

Residential therapy programs provide individuals with brain injury the individualized training and support they need to live in their own homes. The goal of residential programs is to assist individuals in acquiring and maintaining daily living skills, including home maintenance, cooking, personal hygiene, shopping and personal finance management. In addition, emphasis is placed on medical stabilization, problem solving, community involvement, stress management, behavior management, and responsible social, financial, and work behaviors.

Assisted Living Facilities

Assisted living facilities offer housing and other services to assist residents such as availability of aides to provide personal care (assistance with bathing, dressing, taking medications, etc.) on-site nursing or medical care, etc.

Continuing Care Retirement Communities

Continuing care retirement communities offer a variety of living options (such as single family dwellings and apartment buildings/condos), as well as medical and nursing services. There is usually a minimum age requirement as they target people of retirement age. These facilities also offer conveniences such as dining, shopping, banking, and recreational facilities.

Independent Living Facilities/Retirement Communities

Retirement communities offer housing for independent adults, plus organized social and recreational programs. Unlike the continuing care retirement communities, they do not always provide health/medical services available on site. To benefit from this type of residential facility, one would need to be relatively independent. However, there are still benefits as they offer meals, transportation, and social activities that can be very good for someone who has suffered a brain injury.

FAMILY AND MEDICAL LEAVE ACT (FMLA)

As noted previously, the need for 24 hour supervision or assistance is required for the vast majority of people who have sustained a severe traumatic brain injury. Additionally, the injured person will not be able to return to work right away. To achieve the goal of returning home, continuing outpatient rehabilitation, and having the needed supervision at home, the patient and/or family members may need to take time off from work. The Family and Medical Leave Act of 1993 is a United States labor law allowing an employee to take unpaid leave because of a serious health condition that makes the employee unable to perform his or her job or care for a sick family member or a new son or daughter (including by birth, adoption, or foster care). The law recognizes the growing needs of balancing family, work, and obligations and promises numerous protections to workers. Some of these protections include:
- Twelve (12) work weeks of leave per twelve (12) months for various reasons such as
    - Caring for the birth, adoption, or foster care placement issues
    - Caring for a sick child, spouse, or parent
    - Being physically unable to perform one's job
- Restoration to the same position upon return to work. If the same position is unavailable, the employer must provide the worker with a position that is substantially equal in pay, benefits, and responsibility.
- Protection of employee benefits even while on leave. An employee is entitled to reinstatement of all benefits to which the employee was entitled before going on leave.
- Protection of the employee to insure that his or her rights under the Act are not interfered with or denied by an employer.

• Protection of the employee from retaliation by an employer for exercising rights under the Act.

Generally, the Act ensures that all workers are able to take extended leaves of absence from work to handle family issues or illness without fear of being terminated from their jobs by their employers or being forced into a lower job upon their return. The leave guaranteed by the act is unpaid and is available to those working for employers with 50 or more employees within a 75-mile radius. In addition, an employee must have worked for the company at least 12 months and 1,250 hours in the preceding 12 months.

DRIVING AFTER A BRAIN INJURY

For most of us, driving is one of the most important day-to-day activities. Driving symbolizes not only convenience, but freedom and independence. Good driving skills require good sensory, perceptual, cognitive, and motor abilities. As a result, a brain injury can affect our ability to be a safe driver by impairing our decision-making skills and our ability to control a vehicle.

A person who has had any type of brain impairment, whether it is a traumatic brain injury, stroke, or disease process that affects the brain, should first discuss with his or her doctor whether it is safe to return to driving. The doctor may require a formal driving evaluation prior to clearing the patient depending upon the specific impairments. Once any legal and medical obstacles that would disqualify someone from driving are overcome, the person with brain injury may be ready to explore the possibility of driving. First, he or she should contact the Department of Motor Vehicles (DMV, also referred to as Motor Vehicle Administration [MVA]) to ask if there is a special office through which persons with medical needs should apply for a license. Sometimes these offices have separate systems in place that make certain allowances (such as issuing one-day permits allowing driving for the purpose of taking the evaluation without first taking the written test) that can be very helpful.

After a brain injury, one may be required to take a comprehensive driving evaluation. If so, obtain a referral from a physician for a comprehensive driving evaluation by a certified driving rehabilitation specialist (CDRS). A doctor who is familiar with brain injury, perhaps the treating physiatrist or neurologist, would be the best person to give the referral.

An evaluation that includes both clinical and on-the-road evaluation is needed to determine if it is safe for a person with brain injury to resume driving. This evaluation can test your vision (visual acuity, peripheral vision, color blindness, sign recognition), perception (visual discrimination, spatial relationships, depth perception), cognition (memory, attention skills, problem-solving skills), functional ability (strength, coordination, range of motion, sensation), and reaction time. Some people are ready to drive within a few months of their injury. Others may not be ready for years. Remember to arrange for appropriate automobile insurance before driving. Keep in mind that in certain situations, if the doctor has not cleared the person to drive and he or she drives anyway, he or she may not be covered by his or her insurance policy.

Driver rehabilitation specialists can be located through the Association of Driver Rehabilitation Specialists (ADED) at www.aded.net or by phone at (318) 257-5055. The local Department of Motor Vehicles can also provide locations for driver rehabilitation.

Driving Alternatives

Returning to driving may not be possible for some individuals after a brain injury, so it is important to locate other transportation options. It may be necessary to rely on family members or friends at least initially after the brain injury. For some, buses, trains, and subway systems may be an option. Many cities have buses with low floor ramps. Lift-equipped buses make it easy for wheelchair and ambulatory riders to get on and off the bus. Priority seating, typically located behind the driver, is also offered on buses for people with disabilities. If a person needs priority seating, it is okay to ask the driver. It is also okay to ask the driver to tell you when you've arrived at your stop. For those who are hearing or visually impaired, most buses have digital signs and audio systems to announce stops, intersections, and transfer points.

Cities with subways and rail systems have handicapped symbols to direct riders to the elevators. Elevators are equipped with security cameras and emergency intercoms to contact the station manager. Lower panels on farecard machines make it easy for wheelchairs riders to buy fares.

Public transportation can pose challenges, however, for people with cognitive impairments that cause difficulty with memory, money management, awareness of time and place, and appropriate social skills. Community services can provide alternative transportation services to people with brain injury, which can include accessible vans and taxi services. Many of these services are free or very inexpensive. Contact your County Office on Disability for transportation options in your area.

BRAIN INJURY SUPPORT GROUPS AND ORGANIZATIONS

Understanding and coping with injuries affecting the brain are difficult and frustrating for individuals and their family and friends. (See Chapter 10 on emotional and family effects.) Many people with brain injury believe they are alone until they find others with similar experiences. By joining a support group, brain injury survivors and/or their families can learn from others who have had similar experiences. These support groups and brain injury organizations can provide support, information, advice, first-hand guidance, and most of all, hope. In addition, these groups often act as advocates, provide educational information, and bring issues of brain injury to public awareness.

Many states have local chapters that are sanctioned affiliates of the Brain Injury Association of America (BIAA). These affiliate organizations operate programs and services that connect survivors of brain injury, their families and friends, healthcare professional and communities. They also offer brain injury support groups for survivors and caregivers. For more information or to find a support group for the survivor or family, contact the national association or the local chapter. The contact information for BIAA is 1-800-444-6443; their website is http://www.biausa.org.

BRAIN INJURY INFORMATION

For additional resources regarding both medical coverage issues as well as general information for survivors of TBI, some excellent resources are the National Resource Directory, the Defense and Veterans Brain Injury Center (DVBIC), the Centers for Disease Control and Prevention (CDC) and brainline.org.

The National Resource Directory connects service members and veterans to support services and resources available across federal, state, and local government agencies. It includes information on veterans' services and benefit organizations; nonprofit, community-based and faith-based organizations; and academic, professional, and philanthropic organizations. You will find information on benefits and compensation; education, training, and employment; family and caregiver support; healthcare services; housing and transportation; and other miscellaneous services and resources. You can access the resource directory at http://www.nationalresourcedirectory.org.

DVBIC specializes in traumatic brain injury and has excellent educational information for patients, caregivers, and clinicians. Their website is http://www.dvbic.org. Brainline.org is a nonprofit web-based organization, which is funded by DVBIC and WETA (a public broadcasting station in Washington, DC) to provide accurate, up-to-date information for patients and caregivers regarding traumatic brain injury. Their website is http://www.brainline.org.

The CDC provides information on all types of brain injury, not just traumatic brain injury. The CDC offers information on stroke, brain tumors, and other disease processes that affect the brain. Their website is http://www.cdc.gov.

KEY POINTS

- There are many resources available for patients and families at the local and federal levels.
- Case managers and social workers are an excellent resource to help locate the appropriate services.
- The internet can provide excellent information on resources for people with brain injuries and their families.

──16──
LIFE AFTER BRAIN INJURY: PERSONAL STORIES OF RECOVERY

As I recover from this life-altering experience, my mantra has become, "I will not be bitter, I will be better." I believe I have developed a stronger character, greater inner strength, and increased mental endurance. —Selina Brisbaji

Strength from a Community of Faith
Rabbi Lynne Landsberg

"The 12-foot patch of black ice had concerned [Ms.] Williams-Barber and her neighbors for several weeks. At 9:30 am, 10 to 15 minutes after a tow truck had removed [the] Mustang [from the first accident], Williams-Barber heard a huge dull thud, ran to open her front door. The driver's side of a 1988 Jeep was smashed against a tree. Williams heard a little boy inside screaming hysterically. 'He was just in dreadful shock,' Williams-Barber said. 'We didn't know if maybe he was bleeding internally. His mother was laying [sic] beside him unconscious. He was totally distraught.'" —*Washington Post,* January 12, 1999.

The distraught child in the newspaper article was my son Jesse, who had just celebrated his eighth birthday. He emerged without serious physical injury. For me, however, it was an altogether different story. The accident left me with a traumatic brain injury (TBI). I was in a coma for six weeks; initially, the doctors at Georgetown University Hospital were unsure whether I'd live. Once I passed the crucial 72-hour mark still alive, they prepared my husband, Dennis, saying that if I did awake, I would not recognize him or our son.

After four weeks at Georgetown University Hospital, while still in a coma, I was moved to National Rehabilitation Hospital (NRH). At NRH, I did slowly awaken, but it was not a classic Hollywood wakeup. It took well over a month for me to go from being able to move my fingers on command to mumbling a word or two. I could not sit up. I could not hold a straw. I could not feel any emotions whatsoever. NRH provided me with multiple therapies, including physical, occupational, speech and neuropsychological. After four months in the hospital, I was finally able to come home. I required 24-hour nursing for almost two years. Years of therapy began with intensive in-home rehabilitation followed by continued visits to NRH.

My therapists helped me understand that people who sustain a TBI have to reestablish pathways from the brain to the body. In order to do this, they have to learn everything all over again. I had to relearn how to walk, relearn how to talk, relearn how to concentrate and read, and relearn how to perform daily activities.

Before the accident my life was very hectic. I've been told that in my former life, I was an effortless multitasker, a fast talker, and a quick thinker. I had speaking engagements across the country and composed my most powerful speeches in airplanes and taxis. In my former life, I was Rabbi Lynne Landsberg. And although I am still Rabbi Lynne Landsberg, the rest has changed.

I've slowly relearned how to live. But the TBI has left me with persistent physical and cognitive challenges. Now, I walk with a cane, require assistance with minor tasks, and I must speak slowly to be understood. For a New Yorker, that is the hardest part.

Before the accident, I spent eight years as the associate director of the RAC, the Religious Action Center of Reform Judaism (Reform Judaism's social justice advocacy office in Washington, D.C.), serving as legislative director and supervisor of the legislative assistants. Then for more than two years I served as the Union of Reform Judaism's Regional Director of the Mid-Atlantic Council (serving some seventy congregations in a six-state area). In both positions, I worked with Reform Jewish congregations, the larger Jewish community and in interfaith settings.

During my years of continued recovery, I have often reflected on how I managed to find the strength, the resilience to rebuild my life. I have identified three ways that my Jewish community, as well as my local neighborhood community, initially supported and fostered my resilience from the day of my accident forward. Over time, these three forms of support morphed. The community's support transformed as I grew from total dependency to the person I am today — a whole person despite my disability.

All religious groups can use these three ways as a model to help people regain themselves. The first way the community reached out to me was through prayer. The second was by visits. And the third was by providing practical support.

Prayers

I am told that throughout my entire hospital stay, many prayers were offered for my healing in synagogues across the country (and in Israel). At my bedside, rabbis, cantors, and laypeople recited or sang psalms and prayers. My brothers, I am told, were moved to tears when my family rabbi, Rabbi Danny Zemel, suggested that perhaps a really familiar prayer tune might somehow seep into my unconscious.

My family's synagogue, Temple Micah of Washington, D.C., held a healing service on my behalf. Though the service was about me, it helped everyone there a great deal by giving them a way to handle their feelings of fear and helplessness.

Not long after the accident, a rabbi I barely knew went online asking our fellow clergy to recite psalms daily on my behalf. A great many people volunteered, and each one of the Hebrew Bible's 150 psalms was assigned. When I came home from the hospital, almost everyone sent me copies of their psalms, along with beautiful, evocative letters.

I do not believe that God discriminates by healing those patients who garner the most prayers. Rather, I believe that prayer strengthens those who pray, thereby enabling them to reach out and help the one who is stricken. It was as if the arms of the Jewish community were wrapped around me, holding me tightly yet lovingly, keeping me in this world.

Attentive Visits

Especially important to me was the presence of my family. Within two hours of the accident, my 80-year-old father was on a plane from West Palm Beach, Florida, to Washington, D.C. He moved into our house and sat in my hospital room every day for the next four months. Knowing that Dad, Dennis, and my two brothers, Jonathan and Michael, were there filled me with warmth. Jesse did not visit until the last few weeks; the doctors felt that an 8-year-old would be traumatized seeing his mother in a coma with a feeding tube in her stomach, a ventilator in her throat, IV tubes in her arms, and a pressure monitor sticking out of her skull.

In the hospital, my room was often full. The hospital lobby attendant who signed in visitors told my father that I often had more visitors than the rest of the patients in the hospital combined! I don't know if my father was giving out free food, but my room was quite lively, regardless of whether I was conscious or unconscious. Friends, colleagues, and loved ones held my hand, told me stories, coaxed me with humor, and included me in their conversations and laughter even when I could not respond. One friend walked into my coma room, bent over my bed, and commanded: "Lynne, wake up! You're missing the Last Call Sale at Neiman's!" Another visitor was a coworker I had visited in a hospital a few years earlier after she had been struck by lightning. I think one of us must have said, "We have to stop meeting like this."

On a Friday afternoon about three months after the accident, board members of the Reform Movement's Mid-Atlantic Council brought a challah (Sabbath bread) to my hospital bedside. They helped me recite the Motzi (the Hebrew prayer over bread), and we ate the challah. It was the first time since my accident that I had said anything in Hebrew. Reciting a prayer in Hebrew, in community, helped me realize later on that during my hospitalizations (and beyond), I had been on the receiving end of the mitzvah (commandment) of bikur cholim, compassionate and involved visitation of the sick.

Each visit diminished my feelings of isolation and affirmed my connection to the world I had known before my brain injury. While I was in the hospital, those who fulfilled this mitzvah brought the world to me. Once I was settled back home, my visitors brought me to the world.

Practical Support

With their very practical support, the Jewish community as well as my neighbors and friends helped deliver my family from the abyss and ushered me into the next stage of recovery: the post-hospital period.

It is the tradition of all religions that people lend their time and talent to help others. Within my religious community, the "caring committee" of my congregation Temple Micah went into action. While I was in a coma, the committee mobilized Temple Micah members to cook Friday night Sabbath dinners for my three guys at home: my dad, my husband, and my son. Every Friday, a member of Temple Micah would deliver a dinner complete with Shabbat essentials: the braided Sabbath bread or challah, Sabbath candles, and wine for the Sabbath blessing. And after I came home, the meals kept coming, until, with tremendous help from my nurse and Dennis, I was able to prepare our family's Sabbath meal. It would be for me a crucial step forward, as well as the first sobering realization that I would never again be able to do things as I had done them before the accident.

When I had been home for about eight months, four mothers who knew me from a synagogue nursery school our children attended together came to visit. They sat with me in my living room and asked if they could help me relearn how to cook. "Relearn?" I exclaimed. "How about you teach me how to cook!"

My culinary teachers arrived every Sunday morning after they dropped their kids off at religious school. Because I couldn't see well, they typed recipes in large bold type, put them into plastic sleeves, and stored them in a binder. Each time they came, they'd add new recipes, writing them in language a recent TBI survivor could follow. (For instance, a meatloaf recipe prescribed: "Mix the following ingredients together in a blender or food processor. You may have to mix them one ingredient at a time—eggs, potato, onion, then ketchup.") The practical support these women, and so many others, freely gave to our family, encompassing everything from running errands to arranging Jesse's play dates, brought me to the point where I could begin to think about becoming a productive person again.

In the winter of 2000, when I could walk, though I was still unsteady, Rabbi David Saperstein, the Director of the RAC, phoned one day to offer to drive me and my nurse to Baltimore for the annual Jewish Council for Public Affairs Plenum. On the way, Rabbi Saperstein made me gasp when he told me, "I want you back at the Religious Action Center as soon as you're ready." The possibility of my returning to the RAC with a TBI seemed inconceivable. Yet the thought of my contributing again to the Jewish community as well as the opportunity to think and learn and become productive was as irresistible as it was frightening.

It took a year before I was physically and cognitively able to tell David that I would return to the RAC. I began working two hours each Monday and Thursday morning. My occupational therapist accompanied me on my first day to set up my workspace. She also explained to David and the senior staff what I could and could not do (yet) and that they should always give me feedback, positive and negative. My first responsibility was to call congregational rabbis and ask them about the state of their synagogue's social action activity and what RAC materials they had found helpful. In order to prepare myself for making the phone calls, I had to write out a script and practice it with my speech therapist.

In September 2001, I received my first opportunity to speak publicly. The Washington Jewish Community Council asked me to deliver a response in honor of my receiving an award for my prior work in social action. The former Lynne Landsberg used to jot down notes for a talk in the cab on the way over to the presentation. Post-accident, the response took me months to write and weeks to practice with my speech therapist.

The fact that the new Lynne Landsberg cannot speak publicly with the ease of the old is just one of a long list of deficiencies caused by my brain injury. I have come to understand that my healing falls into two categories. In Hebrew, the first is called *rifuat ha nefesh* or a healing of the *nefesh* (commonly translated as soul), and the second is known as *rifuat ha goof,* or healing of the body.

For me, the healing of the body has come far more quickly than my doctors had forecast. But my healing of the soul has been much slower. I think of *goof* as the outer self and *nefesh* as the thinking, feeling, inner self, and I wonder, what does it take to heal the all-encompassing soul?

I know that healing of the *nefesh* requires one to accept certain harsh realities. Continued healing is dependent on my emotional ability to mourn the old Lynne Landsberg and to embrace the slowly developing skills of the new Lynne Landsberg. No longer do I measure my successes by comparing them to my former achievements. It cannot be a matter of what I've lost, but what I've gained: an understanding of how much good is in each and every day and each and every person. And I am thrilled every time I can do something new. Nine years ago it was new for me to be able to smile. Now, I can easily write and deliver a speech. It seems my recovery continues, albeit at a slower pace, but it continues nevertheless. I have also found a satisfying role for the new

Lynne Landsberg — as an advocate for Americans with disabilities. It seems that my activist gut was one organ unaffected by my accident.

When I reentered the world I was shocked at what I learned. *Before* my injury, I belonged to one minority that was cohesive, strong, and articulate and *definitely* heard—the American Jewish community. What I learned was that I now belong to a second minority that is *daily* the victim of discrimination. Although about ten times larger than the American Jewish community, *this* minority remains almost invisible and barely heard; Americans with disabilities. In my former life, when I was the Associate Director of the Religious Action Center, I worked on behalf of the Reform Movement along with other advocates in the interfaith community on a huge new bill that I *never*, in my wildest dreams, thought would directly affect *my* life. In 1990, we helped pass the Americans with Disabilities Act, now known as the ADA.

The ADA is often referred to as the civil rights bill for people with disabilities. Last year, 2008, our country marked the 18th anniversary of the ADA. As a rabbi with a disability, the 18th anniversary, the *"Chai"* anniversary, held special meaning for me. The ADA literally gave new life to Americans with disabilities by altering public physical barriers, making discrimination illegal, and creating new opportunities for education and employment.

Today I am the Senior Advisor on Disability Issues for the Union for Reform Judaism's (URJ) Department of Jewish Family Concerns and the Religious Action Center of Reform Judaism. I work to raise awareness of the needs, both physical and emotional, of people with disabilities within the Jewish community, other religious communities, and the larger American population The URJ is forging ties with other disability activists nationwide and working for the civil and human rights of people with disabilities.

The former Lynne Landsberg was always a political activist, but the new Lynne Landsberg wants to not only change policy, but also change attitudes. The ADA mandates access to public places, but it cannot mandate access to the human heart.

When I walk into meetings, social situations, and commercial establishments with a cane, people often ignore me. However, when I attend disability-related meetings or activities, people don't even see the cane. They just see Lynne Landsberg, and I am invited to participate as a whole person. This is the deepest desire of the disability community: to have people see past the disability and acknowledge the person first.

I know how far my recovery has come from those devastating first months in 1999. And as my family and I continue toward the unknowable future, I understand that the support of my religious community and our neighbors and friends will continue to be there. I understand personally what the Jewish community's respect and inclusion mean for a person with a disability. I know I received access to religious life, and to life in general, not necessarily available to most people with disabilities.

In turn, my greatest wish is to take what I've learned from my experience and sound a wake-up call to the whole religious community that people with disabilities are out there and they need our active involvement. We must break down the physical, communicative, and attitudinal barriers wherever they exist. We must come together and help all Americans recognize that people with disabilities are people first, people with unlimited potential who are not to be defined by their disabilities.

Learning to Live with the Unexpected
Sharon Douglas

It was 4 a.m. on March 24, 2007. It's a date and time I'll never forget. I woke up to the sound of the ringing phone. My husband Fred called me from his security job. "I've got a terrible headache," he told me. He was going to call an ambulance. He was concerned about his car and asked me to come get it. I called our son Ricky and when we were told Fred had been sent to Southern Maryland Hospital, I sent Ricky home. Thinking this was just some minor issue, I followed my husband to the hospital.

When I arrived, Fred was still in agonizing pain. Even the morphine wasn't helping to ease it. I was told that a CT scan showed a bleed on his brain, but they couldn't tell us much more than that. He needed to be transferred to a facility that could really help him, so they decided to get him to the Washington Hospital Center.

Everything seemed to conspire against the transfer. It was cloudy and rainy that day, and the helicopter couldn't get up in the air. He had to be transported on the ground, a trip that would take two hours because there was an annual marathon race in Washington, D.C. that made travel difficult. I went ahead in my car, only to discover that he was being admitted to Georgetown University Hospital. I was just relieved that he was in a place where he could get the help he needed. Fred was in and out of consciousness that day, but tests showed that he had a brain aneurysm positioned behind his left eye that had ruptured. At least we had an answer. Surgery followed, but Fred didn't wake up. He was in a coma for 31 days.

When I'm asked how I got through those days of his silence and unresponsiveness, I always answer with the simple word: "Faith." I prayed. I believed he would wake up. He had to wake up. We have a new baby coming—a grandson and Fred needed to see him. After all, this would be our first grandchild.

So every day I would wake up while it was still dark and leave my home in Bowie, Maryland, at 5 a.m. to arrive at the hospital by 7 a.m. I sat with him talking and reading and behaving as if he could hear everything I said. Then at 1 p.m., I left him to go to work as a Deputy U.S. Marshall. And then I went home again to do the same thing the next day. When I felt sad or overwhelmed, I took refuge in my car and the miles I traveled each day. Cars are a perfect place to cry, I discovered.

Fred and I have been together for more than 30 years. I am his wife. I had to be there even though I wasn't sure if he knew I was there or not. Before his aneurysm, we had never been apart for one night in all our years together. We met on the job as D.C. police officers and have been with each other ever since.

Our children, family, and friends visited, too, keeping his room filled with conversation and laughter. Then one day he woke up. I wasn't there, but it didn't matter. He was back to me, and that was everything. I looked familiar to him, but at first he really didn't know who I was. And he wasn't responding the way he should have. He couldn't walk or sit up. He needed rehabilitation, but if he didn't show some progress, he would end up in a nursing home.

In the early 1990s, I had spent several years working in medical records at the National Rehabilitation Hospital (NRH). I knew that is where Fred needed to be. So I pushed him, and he showed some progress. After weeks at Georgetown, he was transferred to NRH.

I discovered that rehabilitation doesn't always move forward in a straight line. After being admitted to NRH, Fred regressed and seemed to lose what he had gained in those last weeks at Georgetown. So I pushed even harder, moving his legs to exercise his muscles. And that wasn't easy. Fred's a big man: 6 feet, 4 inches to my 5 feet, 7 inches. "You are going to show these people what you can do," I told him. "If you don't, they will send you to a nursing home." I reminded him of a facility close to our home. We would often drive past it to see the residents sitting in wheelchairs outside watching life passing them by. We promised each other that would never happen to us.

I asked questions of all the doctors and nurses. I was told that it would take some time for all the blood in Fred's brain to be absorbed by his body. When that happened, he would begin to heal. They were right.

A couple of weeks after he entered NRH, a nurse told me that when she asked Fred who I was, he had answered, "My spouse." Anyone who knows Fred recognized his classic response! Shortly afterwards, I was startled by the ringing of my home phone one morning at 1 a.m. The caller ID showed "NRH," and my first thought was that something bad had happened. To my surprise it was Fred, and his first question to me was, "Why did you put me in the hospital?" After getting over the shock and elation of hearing his voice for the first time in two months, I told Fred what had happened to him weeks before and explained the details of the previous two months' events. He remembered very little, and what he did remember was just a vague recollection.

He was beginning to make his way back, but it was the music of Fred's favorite Motown group that really seemed to make a real difference to his recovery. A therapist recommended that I bring in CDs for Fred to listen to as a way to help improve his communication skills. So I flooded his room with the Temptations' music and sang along. Pretty soon, Fred was joining in. He was singing "My Girl" before he really started talking very much.

The music did the trick. Singing seemed to encourage his speech, and he began to talk more and more. He knew me, and he then recognized pictures of our son Ricky and daughter Ryan. And finally, we showed him photos of his newest grandson, Royal, born to our son and daughter-in-law while Fred was in his coma. Then he held Royal on his lap in his wheelchair, and that's when we knew he would really return to us.

Still, these were very scary times, but I took those feelings home with me away from Fred. I listened to music, too, singing in the car on the way home. My family was wonderfully supportive through these difficult times.

After two months at NRH, Fred came home. Then outpatient therapy followed. In October 2007, just seven months after he was close to death, he was able to watch the birth of our second grandchild, a little girl, Anaiah, born to our daughter, Ryan. Ryan asked her Dad to be with her to witness this amazing miracle.

Now two years later, Fred is just about his old self again. His body is strong, and his speech is fine. He does have some cognitive problems and is blind in his left eye, with limited vision in his right. He has some problems with seizures when he is fatigued and isn't able to return to work. Because I have to work, Ryan stays at home to watch over Fred. It's a sacrifice, but she's Daddy's girl and wants to be there for him. Fred loves his granddaughter and gets to spend hours each day with her.

How can a family survive this kind of devastating event? *Be there*. Don't give up. *Ask questions* and find answers in books and on the Internet. When I knew what happened to Fred, I read all I could about brain aneurisms. I read blogs written by families. I never wanted to feel that I would just accept whatever I was told. I needed to learn all I could so I could help as much as I could. I needed to know what to expect when I got home and how to handle and deal with most situations, such as medications, daily activities, and how to help Fred get reacquainted with family life and our home, even the dogs.

Be a hard taskmaster when it's needed. Sometimes I found I needed to push Fred a bit harder to force him to learn to do things for himself. "I'm not going to feed you. You need to pick up the fork and feed yourself," I would say. "Don't sit in the wheelchair. Stand up and try to walk." And it worked. But to every taskmaster there must be a softer, gentler side. So there would be times on a Saturday or Sunday (after church) when I would wheel him to the solarium at the hospital and give him a pedicure and manicure, and bring him a favorite food. Every day, I would wheel him through the hospital garden so he could feel the fresh air and sunshine.

There is no question that this experience has changed our family. We are a kinder, gentler family now. Knowing that at any second everything in your life can change makes you more aware of each other, more respectful of feelings. The unexpected can happen, we have learned. At 10 p.m. one night I said good-bye to my husband and hours later, he called me to tell me he was dying. He is here now, and we are together more connected than ever before.

Reworking the Grand Plan
Brian Mosko

I was on the job one day in March 2008 when I tumbled from a large trash container and sent my life spinning. I fell against two containers, striking my head at the back and front. I have no memory of what happened next. I was in and out of consciousness. Luckily I was found by some workers on the scene, and I had identification in my wallet. I was rushed to the hospital and my wife, Jenifer, was notified.

I had a closed head injury, and while I looked relatively physically fit, my brain had suffered from the assault. I'm told I was agitated and angry, pulling at my IV and trying mightily to get out of bed, to get out of there. After a week in the intensive care unit (ICU), I had made some progress and began to understand where I was. By the end of the second week, I recognized most of what the people around me were saying, but it was clear that my speech was impaired.

As a top-earning sales rep for a large, national pest management company, I relied on my wits and my easy way with words to meet with clients and seal the deal. Suddenly I was unsure and confused. I couldn't find the right words to say, a language recall problem I now know is common in head injuries of my kind.

After two weeks in acute care, I transferred to the National Rehabilitation Hospital (NRH). But all I really wanted to do was go home to my wife, son Alex and daughter Caroline. I just wanted everything to be as it had been. My first clear words after two weeks were a proclamation to my wife: "I'm not staying here!"

I was very motivated to get back to the "normal" Brian, the familiar Brian, and the Brian at ease with the world, with words, with the life I had built with Jenifer. We met in college and have been together ever since. I studied education and psychology. In school, Jenifer was always amazed that I could pull together a presentation at the last minute, deliver it flawlessly in front of a university classroom, and score a decent grade. After I graduated I taught school, commanding the attention of a classroom full of elementary age children. Now I couldn't string together a coherent sentence, but I was determined to be myself again—the old articulate Brian.

True to my first words, I was out of NRH in fast order. I worked hard to get myself physically well. Two weeks of lying in a bed had taken its toll, so I walked laps around the gym at the hospital, worked out with equipment, and exercised all day long. I was feeling strong, but in speech therapy, I was having difficulty identifying kindergarten-level words from flash cards. So I continued therapy on an outpatient basis at a program close to home.

Three times a week for three months I went to both speech and physical therapies. By the end of June, I had progressed as far as conventional speech therapy could take me. Still I needed more. I'm the head of the household and needed to get back to work. So I began working with Neuropsychologist Dr. Penny Wolfe to push beyond that threshold and deal with the frustration that continues to accompany my recovery. I'm making progress, but I have not gotten back the fluidity of speech I had before. By July 2008, I began going into my office just for a few hours a week. I knew I needed to get into some type of routine to break the frustration and boredom that I was feeling.

I have had enormous support from coworkers and bosses, who have given me a wide berth in which to recover. Still I know that it may be difficult for some people to understand what has happened to me. I don't look any different. I don't have any physical scars from my injury. They can't see the jumble of words in my brain that I have to unscramble before speaking. They can't see the pain I feel as if my brain were pressing hard against my skull. It is hard to see the sleeplessness, the sensitivity to light and noise, or the gastrointestinal problems that have resulted from medications I take to control seizures and pain.

I'm trying to learn to think and speak in a more precise and methodical way. Instead of speaking before I think—which was my common practice—I now have to move slowly across my memory to seek out words and then verbalize my thoughts. There has been improvement, but I am not yet myself. I realize I may never be able to rebuild that old and quick-witted speech pattern. The cells in the speech area of the brain are rebuilding slowly, I'm told. I want them to hurry up and do their job!

While my employer has been flexible, and my wife and I had disability insurance to supplement my income, there are financial constraints. We have had to change the way we live. Jenifer is studying for a graduate degree and hopes to go back to work. Before the accident, we had a plan. With my more flexible schedule I would be able to be at home to meet my kids after school and Jenifer would get them off to school. Now we know we may have to rework the grand plan.

Today I am back to work short hours, three days a week and volunteering in my daughter's kindergarten class as well. Still nearly a year after the injury, work and play can be taxing and tiring.

My wife, my children, and I have had to adjust to a very different life than the life we had before. In our 16 years together, Jenifer and I have had to face some difficult times: a diagnosis of Asberger syndrome for our 8-year-old son Alex and a very serious infection that threatened 5-year-old Caroline. The brain injury has been another real challenge that is testing our family, but I have always been very determined and that hasn't changed. We are working together to push past it as a family and get our lives back in order. While it may be a different, slightly reconfigured life, I'm highly motivated to make it a rich and rewarding one for all of us.

My Soldier's Keeper
Lorrie Knight-Major

Ryan graduated from high school in 2003. Like a lot of young men, he wasn't sure what career path to follow, but after long conversations with family, friends, and an Army recruiter, he decided to dedicate his life to serving his country. He loved being a soldier then and still does. He trained diligently to be the best possible soldier he could be. When it came time for him to begin his tour in Iraq, he was proud to serve to defend the United States. He wanted nothing more than to be a great soldier and leader.

When you have a child serving in a combat zone, the worst nightmare possible is a phone call from the military. At 12:15 p.m. on Friday, November 10, after wrapping up a three-day business meeting in Virginia, I checked my cell phone messages. "This is Sgt 1st Class Williamson with the United States Army," a voice said. "I am calling in regard to your son, Ryan Major. Please call me." Before his second sentence was completed, the tears were flowing down my face. I didn't have the strength to return the call. I ran back to the conference room where my boss, Nicole, was still sitting. I tried to tell her what I had just heard, but I struggled to make myself understood. Somehow I gained enough composure to tell her about the message. I said that the U.S. Army only calls loved ones for one of three reasons: 1) Your son has been killed; 2) Your son has been severely injured; or 3) Your son is missing in action.

Any of these three scenarios was frightening beyond comprehension.

Nicole called Sgt. Williamson back for me and put the phone on speaker. The Sgt. described what had happened. Ryan's unit was on foot patrol in Ramadi, Iraq, when an improvised explosive device was detonated within two feet of where Ryan stood. Ryan was critically wounded. As he listed Ryan's injuries, I cried hysterically on the floor. Nicole took the phone off speaker and finished speaking to Sgt. Williamson outside of the room.

There were many casualties in his unit, but Ryan's injuries were by far the worst: his right leg had already been amputated; he had severe injuries to his right pelvis and burns to his left leg and arms; both his arms were fractured; and there were other internal injuries and a probable traumatic brain injury (TBI), which could not be assessed until he came out of the coma.

My older son, Michael, and I met Ryan at his bedside in the intensive care unit in Landsthul, Germany, three days after I had received the news. When we arrived at Landsthul Hospital, we were met by a team of doctors and clergy. Before taking us to Ryan's room, they escorted us to a chapel. I wanted desperately to see Ryan, but I resisted the desire. I was afraid that they were leading us to the chapel to inform us that Ryan was brain dead.

One of the doctors spoke and told us that they needed to make sure we understood the seriousness of Ryan's injuries. I told them that I was a nurse and showed them the notebook I had prepared with all the information the medical staff had shared by phone during the past few days. The doctors treating Ryan did not believe he would survive.

Like any good nurse, I asked the doctor for the data. "What were the stats of Ryan's survival?" The odds weighed heavily against him. "There is a 70-percent chance that he won't survive," he told me. "That 70-percent chance is gaining on us," I said, "because you are all in here with us and not at Ryan's bedside treating him." I asked them to do their very best to stabilize him so that he could be transferred to the United States. "I did not come to Germany to bring my son back in a body bag."

For the first time in my life, I faced one of my children with multiple traumas, badly disfigured, slipping away—dying. As I approached Ryan's hospital room, I could see him through the glass walls. He was difficult to recognize because his entire body was swollen, but through all of the tubes and machines, I could see my son—in a coma and unable to breathe on his own, but he was there, none the less.

He was connected to a ventilator that breathed for him. There was a feeding tube threaded through his nose and into his stomach. An endotracheal tube went down to his lungs through his mouth. His eyes were closed and were oozing clear lubricant that the nurses continually applied to keep them moist. There was a chest tube in his left lung because of a pneumothorax. His arms and legs were bandaged over wounds that continually oozed. Then there was a catheter for urine and stool. An IV line was in his chest to continuously infuse blood into his veins in order to keep pace with tremendous amounts of blood he continued to lose from his wounds. The only body parts that were spared from the blast were his face, neck, and chest.

I was frightened beyond description; but as bad as Ryan looked, I knew in my heart, he was a fighter. As a child, he had challenged every line I had drawn in the sand. Now I was certain that determination would save his life. Even though he lay there helpless, I believed that if given a fighting chance and the best possible medical care available, Ryan would persevere.

Within 24 hours of our arrival in Landsthul, doctors had stabilized Ryan for transport to Walter Reed Army Medical Hospital in Washington, D.C. I was allowed to fly with Ryan back to Andrews Air Force Base where a Walter Reed Hospital ambulance bus was waiting to transport Ryan and other injured soldiers.

It was just four days since he had been injured in Iraq. He was still in a coma and fighting for his life. He was being treated for multiple infections. We still didn't know if Ryan would survive. And, if he did survive and wake up from the coma, we didn't know what kind of serious or permanent damage the TBI may have caused.

There isn't anything that prepares a mother for the news that her child has suffered life-threatening traumas and, most likely, a serious brain injury. As a nurse, the brain injury was the most difficult to imagine because I had taken care of patients with TBI, and I knew the enormous challenges that patients, families, and caregivers face.

Some of Ryan's doctors tried to be encouraging and optimistic. His coma was medically induced, they told us. Once the heavy pain medications were removed, some of the doctors believed Ryan might wake up, but it was touch and go for the first eight weeks. It was nearly as long before his physicians were certain the rampant infections that had accompanied his injuries were under control.

Three weeks after he was put into the coma, Ryan woke up. While that was more than two years ago, I can visualize the moment as vividly as if it had happened yesterday. Everyone was excited. The problem was, Ryan was awake but was not speaking. Not a sound came out of his mouth. His eyes would sometimes follow me as I moved around his room, but not all the time. While I tried to be optimistic, I often feared the worst.

A few days after he had awakened, Ryan spoke his first word: "No." I had asked him if he could blink his eyes. I sat patiently as he forced the word out of his mouth and as he put the emphasis on the "*n*."

That first word opened a floodgate of words. Ryan was completely uninhibited and verbalized whatever he was feeling. He cussed like a sailor. I had never heard Ryan use foul language before, and for the next 72 hours, his vocabulary was filled with expletives. I was afraid that my son's head injury was so severe that it had left him completely unaware of socially acceptable behavior. I recall thinking to myself, if this was the "new" Ryan, I would prefer that the doctors put him back to sleep! Fortunately for us, this behavior was short-lived, lasting all of 72 hours and never rearing its ugly head again.

Despite those odd few days of uncharacteristic behavior, I was elated that Ryan had awakened and was speaking. One of his first requests was, "I want some Aquafina." It seemed an odd way to ask for water, and not at all like Ryan. Then I noticed a bottle of Aquafina water that I had been drinking sitting on the bedside table. Later that day, his friend Cory came to visit and was drinking a Coke. So Ryan asked for some Coca-Cola. When he watched commercials for fast food restaurants on television, he would ask for the food items by name. I was happy to hear him talk, but disappointed that I couldn't indulge him since he was being fed a liquid diet through his nose and was not allowed to eat.

Days later, Ryan asked his brother Michael to take him home. Michael tried to explain to Ryan that he was very sick and needed to be in the hospital. Ryan repeatedly demanded that Michael pick him up and carry him out of the hospital. It was heartbreaking to listen to his pleas, and while we tried to reason with Ryan, he didn't and couldn't understand.

Ryan didn't realize the gravity of his injuries – a common effect of brain injury. He was so weak he wasn't even able to lift his head off of the pillow. He couldn't move any of his fingers. He could only blink his eyes and turn his head slightly to the left and right, but that didn't stop him from asking several of his male friends to pick him up and take him home.

Ryan's hospital course at Walter Reed was a roller coaster ride of highs and lows. There were frequent setbacks because of infections, heart malfunctioning, electrolyte imbalances, and intestinal illnesses. Ultimately, a second leg amputation was performed because of a serious infection.

Fighting for the Best

In mid-December, Ryan was nearly stable enough to be transferred to a rehabilitation hospital. We were given four options of VA hospitals in the United States, but none was close to home. Ryan's transfer to any of them would require me to travel out of state and live for many months far from home, social support, and my job, and leaving my minor child at home.

My family and friends began working diligently investigating rehab hospitals close to our Silver Spring, Maryland, home and I toured a few of them. One of them was the National Rehabilitation Hospital (NRH), just 16 miles from our house. NRH is one of the top 10 rehabilitation hospitals in the United States. After a tour of the hospital, I decided that it was the best place for Ryan. I was impressed. The facility was beautiful. The staff was warm and friendly. There was a dedicated TBI unit with very knowledgeable and well-trained staff, but getting Ryan into NRH wasn't easy because he is an enlisted soldier. It took some arm twisting and multiple meetings with military staff; ultimately, they granted permission. I convinced them that NRH had a proven track record and that Ryan's family and friends could routinely visit. I felt this support would be critical to his successful recovery.

A week before Ryan's scheduled transfer, he took a turn for the worse. On December 29, 2006, after routine surgery, tissue samples taken during the procedure showed life threatening fungal infection tissue present in his abdominal wound. Another surgery was ordered to remove any abdominal tissue that didn't look healthy. I spoke to the doctors caring for Ryan and requested his transfer to the University of Maryland Medical System (UMMS) Shock Trauma Center. This center is world renowned for managing difficult traumas and complicated infections. It is the only free-standing hospital center in the world dedicated to trauma. I simply wanted the best for my son, and once again, I won the battle with military command. On January 3, 2007, Ryan was moved by ambulance to UMMS Shock Trauma Center. It proved to be a very painful ride because of a dangerous and large bed sore that nearly covered the entire sacral area (the lower back) and reached into the bone. While he had previously been treated with narcotics, he had had little relief from the pain.

Within hours of Ryan's admission to UMMS Shock Trauma Center, the pain team was on board employing its unique holistic approach to treatment. The team used a host of tools including narcotics, Reike therapy, massage therapy, and, later, acupuncture. For the first time in three weeks, Ryan was able to sleep through the night peacefully, as the staff turned him every two hours.

Both Ryan and I will forever be grateful for the healing power of Reike therapy. It works by empowering patients through their active participation in the healing process. On a subsequent admission to UMMS Shock Trauma Center a few months later, Ryan told Bonnie, the Reike Master, "The doctors gave me back my body, but Reike gave me back my soul." Reike has had a profound effect on Ryan, and I credit it with helping him wean completely off narcotic pain medications in less than a year. The doctors and pain team not only successfully treated the fungal infection that had ravaged his body, but also they began the critical restoration of his spirit. Ryan steadily improved, and after one month, he was transferred to NRH where he blossomed.

The Rehabilitation Process

Ryan's transition to NRH was initially very scary for him. He feared being alone at night. He was afraid of the dark. He was still having nightmares about the explosion. He often tried to keep me by his side and delay my going home by asking me do small chores in his room. Ryan's friends and I stayed overnight with him regularly, but we could not stay every night. While at Walter Reed and UMMS Shock Trauma Center, Ryan had never slept alone. His fears were common symptoms of traumatic brain injury and of post-traumatic stress disorder and now both diagnoses were confirmed.

The NRH staff was very aware of Ryan's fear and provided an overnight attendant who stayed inside Ryan's door, allowing Ryan to

sleep at night with the lights out. The nursing staff was very cog-
nizant of Ryan's difficulties and gave him additional attention to
help alleviate his fears.

Ryan's primary reason for transferring to NRH was for rehabilitation and their experience in TBI. Therapy began even before Ryan
could leave his bed. Still one of the first priorities was getting the
skin wound healed. The wound care nurse was very proactive. She
had arranged for the appropriate bed to be in Ryan's room upon his
arrival and developed a comprehensive care plan that included
weekly rounds to assess the wound and weekly photos to assess
improvement.

Ryan had an array of therapies including physical, occupational,
speech, and cognitive therapy. All were grueling for Ryan. He
thought his therapists were giving him too much work. He com-
plained daily about the speech therapist's complex homework
assignments of real world tasks, such as completing Internet
research projects, planning trips, obtaining hospital patient counts
from the various inpatient units, and finally, preparing a Powerpoint
presentation. Initially, Ryan struggled, but as time progressed, the
work got easier. Ultimately, Ryan was able to see the benefits of his
hard work. All the therapy helped Ryan build his strength. Now he
believes it was the speech therapy that played a large role in
improving his cognitive abilities, and for that he will always be
grateful.

Finding a good psychologist is challenging in any environment,
and I was very concerned that Ryan would have trouble opening up
to one. The first psychologist he talked with wasn't a good match.
She recognized this and referred Ryan to a male colleague and former member of the military. He was a perfect fit. While it is very
difficult for most 22-year-olds to discuss their fears and personal
concerns with strangers, Ryan believes this experience helped him
face and accept what had happened to him.

All of Ryan's therapists had an enormous job to do. They had to
challenge him, but remain constantly aware of his fragile emotional
state. They did that with ease. Ryan was committed to getting better, and they were dedicated to helping him achieve his goal.
Through his rehabilitation, Ryan regained his confidence and grew
to know that he could deal with the challenges of being a disabled
person.

American Volunteerism

I knew that the time would come quickly for my son to transition home. I didn't know how I would accomplish the huge task of making our home wheelchair accessible. I was given a 10-page typed list of non-profit groups that might be of assistance. Out of a list of over 140 organizations, countless phone calls, and emails, only one group returned my phone call and provided assistance: the Yellow Ribbon Fund. The Yellow Ribbon Fund was instrumental in providing a rental van for the weekend on short notice, which allowed me to take Ryan home for his first overnight visit while still a patient at NRH.

Fortunately, I learned by word of mouth about "Rebuilding Together Montgomery County," an organization that immediately committed to complete the renovations that would make our home accessible to Ryan. This project was not just about installing an elevator or renovating the bathroom or adding a new deck. It was a life-changing experience. Without the modifications, Ryan would be confined to the basement apart from his family or dependent on his brothers and friends to carry him up and down the stairs. The elevator and handicap accessibility renovations give Ryan the freedom and independence to move around his home.

Lessons Learned

The road to recovery has been an arduous one, paved with many frustrations, disappointments and medical setbacks. There are a few things I wish I had known two years ago:

- Accept help from people. Make it easy for them. Many of your family members, friends, and community will want to support you, but may not know how. Tell them what you need, such as food shopping, providing some hot meals, or taking care of home office duties like writing checks for bills.
- Get a day planner with a business card holder. There will be many times during the acute phase of the injury in which you may be approached by organizations offering assistance. You may not be mentally or emotionally ready to receive the information. Take their cards and make notations. Write the date that you met each person and what services that they provide on the card. You will

have the information available when you actually need it.

• Keep a notebook binder to maintain the medical information and include information about the diagnosis, treatment, physicians, and medications.

• Write your medical questions down so that when the physician stops by the room, you will have all of your questions answered. Restate to the doctor what you believe he or she had told you to be certain you understand correctly.

• Consider individual psychotherapy for caregivers and other family members. This time is very stressful, and it affects everyone.

I have so many blessings for which to be thankful. Most importantly, I'm thankful to God for saving my son's life against enormous odds and for bringing so many caring and generous people into our lives.

Ryan will require several more surgeries over the next two years. Yet, every day he gets better and stronger and more confident about his future plans. He knows there will be obstacles and setbacks along the way, but he is more determined than ever to move forward. Ryan continuously challenges himself. In just the last year, he completed three races using a hand crank bike: the Hope and Possibility 5K Run, the Army 10 Miler, and the New York Marathon. Ryan plans to attend college and major in business administration. Today he is completing the necessary nonprofit 501(3)C paperwork to establish the Sgt. Ryan Major Foundation to provide financial assistance to other military families. Last year, Ryan and two grade school friends started a business, Major Scanning Business Solutions, which provides corporate document management.

Ryan and I know that his continued recovery could not be possible without the prayers, assistance and support of countless people: medical staff, family, friends, volunteers, Veterans support organizations, and the kindness of countless strangers. Ryan's quest for a productive life has been possible only because of the generosity, time, and efforts of the community.

There is a famous quotation by, Orison Swett Marden, that has been our family motto: "Success is not measured by what you accomplish, but by the opposition you have encountered and the courage with which you have maintained the struggle against overwhelming odds." That's a lesson we have all learned. Today, I can proudly say that my son is one of the most successful people I have ever known. Ryan is my hero.

My Eyes, Your Eyes
Selina Brijbasi and Myrtle Brijbasi

My Eyes: Selina

January 5, 2007, was an affirmation of my belief in divine intervention because I ended up in the right place at the right time. Had I not been surrounded by knowledgeable, thoughtful, and caring healthcare professionals with whom I worked, I might not have survived to tell my story. The past two years have been very interesting to say the least. It has been a roller coaster ride like no other. A catastrophic brain injury, multiple surgeries, extended hospital stays, aggressive therapies to achieve set goals, a faith journey, and having to relearn everything to become independent again, have been a transformation of trials into triumphs.

Five days into 2007, my seemingly successful workday as an occupational therapist was suddenly interrupted with an intense headache. Minutes later, I lost consciousness. On that day, I suffered a devastating ateriovenous malformation (AVM) rupture, collapsed, and ended up having emergency brain surgery to remove a massive hematoma. I was completely unresponsive. Machines monitored any and all signs of my life for days following surgery. One week later, my night nurse recorded that I responded to her command to lift my index finger. This was welcoming news to everyone including doctors, nurses, other medical caregivers, family and friends. That moment marked the beginning of a long road to recovery, more surgeries, therapy, and rehabilitation. Even though I became more and more alert and was recognizing people around me, I was imprisoned in my own body. I could not speak, move on my own, breathe independently, nor express my thoughts. I cried and frowned more than I smiled because I was so frustrated that I could not verbally communicate with the people by my bedside. I could only respond with thumbs-up gestures and eye blinks. Nevertheless, I felt the love and heard the many prayers and the inspirational words from cards that were read to me. I enjoyed the soothing music that played, and yes, I also tuned in and out to the up-to-the-minute news that my friends, family, and visitors shared with me. I was thankful, but yet very helpless, in expressing that thankfulness. I prayed too, asking God to help me become well again, so that I could one day express that thankfulness myself, and let everyone know what I was experiencing.

Finally, I can do that. I am thankful to God for my recovery thus far. I am also thankful to all the medical personnel who attended to my needs and provided the medical treatments and therapies that were warranted. To my family and friends, I am totally indebted for your love and dedication. I can now speak, read, and laugh with as much enthusiasm and mental sharpness as ever. I can even use the computer, my favorite cognitive engagement, and I enjoy participating in the game of "Taboo" with family and friends. I also enjoy the outdoors again. Attending church service, especially at Christmas, Easter, and other special services, has been overwhelming and full of precious moments. To my church family, you were the pillar of strength for me and my family. Hospital visits from my pastor and lay visitor were also moments that reinforced the powerful nature of God and how He directs our paths as Christians. Without prior notice, they were often present at my bedside on a day that I was either having a major or a minor medical procedure, or was engaged in therapy sessions that marked a milestone in my recovery. These visits were a most remarkable and a boost to my faith journey. Through continuous prayer, I have learned to be patient on the Lord and to believe in possibilities.

Two years later, my medical checkup with my neurosurgeons was very positive, and I have been released from their care. All of my MRIs were clear. I am alive and healthy. I have a wonderful family and great friends. With the Lord by my side, and my total commitment to strive for independence through my therapy sessions, I will achieve my ultimate goal, which is to be totally rehabilitated and return to work.

I am grateful for many things. Among these are the journals that were kept for me by friends and family. They helped me to realize many things, but most importantly, they helped me realize how profound well wishes, prayers, and words of encouragement can be. On the cover of one of the two journals, a friend made for me, were the wonderful words: "May this book be filled with encouragement, inspiration, and love for Selina! However you feel led, please share a few words. I hope that these messages can motivate Selina along her recovery and life!"

The wonderful accounts in the journals allowed me to experience in real time what I can't recall so I have not missed out on anything. I was also made aware of the milestones I overcame along the way. The journals helped me to place events, days, dates, and months in perspective. Through these writings, I also realized how much my injury affected family and friends, and learned just how many other people's lives I touched and inspired more than I ever had been aware.

The journals were a phenomenal demonstration of love, support, encouragement, and the power of prayer from my cheerleaders: family, friends, caregivers, church family, and everyone's extended families who became engaged in prayer chains from all over the world. This testament of faith further strengthened my spirituality and helped me to adopt a very positive attitude.

One day, while listening to one of Joel Osteen's televised sermons, he referenced the statement, "A setback is a setup for a greater comeback." I was totally intrigued by these words, and after some time of internalizing, I understood their truth. I told myself that I will not see my circumstances as a set of limitations. Instead, I will see my experience as one that has given me the tools to thrust me forward in all aspects of life.

I have since developed a greater appreciation for my being, and I am reminded not to take anything for granted. I also concluded that just because a person has been affected by life-changing events and may not often feel "normal," one can still maintain an integral role in society by participating in a myriad of social and recreational activities organized by family, friends, caregivers, and adaptive recreational sports organizations.

For me, participation in these activities allowed me to demonstrate my independence and helped me to recognize just how far I have traveled on the road to recovery. Among these activities have been day trips to places of interest such as galleries, public libraries, museums, and open air markets; musical theaters, concerts, bingo, and friend and family functions; visiting malls and shopping centers; and weekend getaways, swimming and skiing. Yes, I can confidently say that I am enjoying an improved, overall quality of life in spite of the fact that I still have some more goals to achieve.

As I recover from this life-altering experience, my mantra has become: "I will not be bitter, I will be better." I believe I have developed a stronger character, greater inner strength, and increased mental endurance. I have recognized the enormity of my emotional growth. Through my spirituality and strengthened faith, my professional life as an occupational therapist now has greater meaning. I can surely empathize with my patients, as I have walked in their shoes. I fully understand their anxieties, their frustrations, and their joys.

One of the journal entries made by a college classmate reminded me of a comment I made in class that I had actually forgotten. "I wondered why I chose to become an OT," I said. That same classmate assured me that my knowledge and skill as an OT was a blessing in disguise, and that coupled with my Christian faith, my health is being restored, and that I am in control of my recovery. This is so prophetic! As an occupational therapist, I have learned that *recovery means living successfully with dysfunction*. I am now experiencing "recovery" and am more appreciative of my calling in life, and my God-given talents, which I have used in the past to assist and enrich the lives of individuals with cognitive and physical impairments.

Throughout my ordeal, I have never asked "Why me?" And I know there is no easy answer to that question. However, what I do know deep down in my heart is that I will use my experience to be an inspiration to my patients. Today, reflecting on my life I can't help but think of these words: "Life threw me a punch to try and knock me out, but as in any good fist fight, the winner gets the last punch. In life, I am still swinging, and still rolling with the punches."

Your Eyes: Myrtle

Being a parent is a beautiful thing. It is every parent's greatest pride to watch their children grow into responsible adults with successful careers. A parent envisions that wonderful future for their children, full of opportunities.

As a parent, you always feel some degree of concern about your children's well-being. Still, never in a million years do you imagine that you will receive a distress call about any of them, but I have experienced all of that joy and pride—as well as that awful nightmare.

At about noon on January 5, 2007, a rainy and wintry day, my phone vibrated as I was on my way to a class in the school where I am a teacher. At the other end of the line was Selina's cheery voice saying, "Hi Mom! Just a reminder that I'll see you later this evening after work."

I hadn't seen her since Christmas and I was looking forward to the visit. The conversation continued. "I have a headache and I am going to rest up before coming home," Selina said. It was a one-hour drive. We ended our conversation with the usual "love you, and see you soon."

Fifteen minutes later my phone vibrated again. Checking on the number, I recognized it was Selina and decided not to answer, but an inner voice said, "Let her know that I cannot speak now and will call later." To my dismay when I answered, it wasn't Selina's voice. Instead, it was a fast-talking, anxious voice of one of her coworkers telling me that Selina had collapsed at work and was being rushed by ambulance to Good Samaritan Hospital in Baltimore, and that the EMT in attendance needed to speak with me regarding insurance and clinical history.

To say the least, the news was shocking. Instantly, I felt shivers throughout my body. Then, I was momentarily paralyzed. My emotions ranged from disbelief, anxiety, confusion, fear, to the "what ifs." By then, I was hyperventilating. I was moving down the school hall but had no feelings in my legs. I felt helpless.

There is definitely no formula to apply in response to such news. As a Christian, I called on God to give me the strength, divine order, and guidance to deal with this situation. My prayer was immediately answered, and from that moment, calm came over me, allowing me to think and act logically.

I was back and forth on the phone with medical personnel providing the information they needed. I called relatives in Baltimore and asked them to get to the hospital as soon as possible, and to act on our behalf until my husband and I could get there. I spoke to some of my colleagues about my family emergency, contacted other family members and my church, and I left for the hospital. Trust me, I prayed without ceasing, not realizing that the worst news was yet to come.

Within minutes of Selina's arrival at the hospital, another call came from her cell phone. This time I am being asked permission by the medical team to perform emergency brain surgery due to an AVM rupture. An impulsive "yes" was my response. Before I could inform them to contact her neurosurgeon, Dr. Nair, whose office is at that hospital, I was being told that he had been called and was en route to perform the surgery. I felt relieved and trusted his medical expertise since he had diagnosed Selina's AVM in 2000, following complaints of severe headaches. Selina had received radiation treatment at Johns Hopkins Hospital for the AVM, and although the treatment was successful, we knew that there was a 2-percent rate of recurrence. Unfortunately, Selina fell among that 2-percent.

Selina's surgery was successful, but the road to recovery was long. Upon arrival at the hospital, my husband and I were able to see her in the recovery room. Dr. Nair explained the details of the surgery and the prognosis. Though we were assured of her recovery, possibilities, and outcomes, the negatives were frightening. I found myself listening to, and praying only for, the positives. After the initial shock of seeing her in the recovery room hooked up to machines and tubes of varying kinds, I was thankful that she was alive. I was also overwhelmed by the outpouring of love and compassion from family, friends, Selina's coworkers, the president of the hospital, my pastor, and lay visitors. Selina was an occupational therapist employed at the Good Samaritan Nursing Center, which is part of the Good Samaritan Hospital network.

Two years later, and after multiple surgeries, lengthy hospital stays, inpatient and outpatient rehabilitation in speech, physical, and occupational therapy, we are truly blessed that Selina is alive. There is no cognitive impairment, and though walking is her greatest challenge, significant improvement is evident.

Selina's illness and recovery have been an extraordinary journey: spiritual, emotional, and physical. Mental toughness amid the "what ifs" and optimism were the attitudes I adopted. Education about Selina's medical condition and the treatments beneficial to her consumed my life. Asking questions and my unwavering commitment to support her, love her, and make the best decisions on her behalf became my new tasks and purpose in life.

I was assertive but professional. I was observant and never timid to ask why. I initiated conversations because I had an insatiable desire for an explanation to everything. Fortunately, the medical professionals with whom I have interacted engaged me in meaningful and informative conversations and provided supplemental literature for me to read. I am most grateful for their cooperation and accommodation.

Throughout Selina's hospitalization and rehabilitation, my respect for medical personnel—the doctors, nurses, therapists, technicians, and all personnel associated with her care—has been elevated to new heights. Everyone who attended to her was genuinely interested in her care and well-being. I appreciated everyone's tenderness and their kind and endearing words. Everyone's politeness and professionalism were remarkable. Everyone who interacted with Selina throughout her illness and recovery today celebrates her successes and encourages her even when progress seems slow. I cannot emphasize enough how heartwarming such acts of compassion have been to Selina and my family. We do feel blessed. Thank you for all that you do to improve the quality of life of our loved ones.

During the long months of recovery, coping mechanisms became the order of the day. I am happy to share the ones that worked for me with everyone whose loved ones are undergoing treatment and rehabilitation for brain injury. I extend my prayers and best wishes to all of you.

- Be prayerful! Rely heavily on your spirituality for strength and divine order in your life throughout the recovery process. Embrace your church family, friends, and prayer partners/circles as they offer prayers for you, your family, and especially your loved one who is ill.
- Condition yourself to exercise extraordinary patience all the time no matter how tired you are. Recovery from brain injury is a lengthy process . . . years.
- Be realistic, remain positive, and give love unconditionally. Become educated about the medical condition and listen well to the medical personnel. Your loved one will always be your major concern.
- Become a pillar of strength because the patient is looking to you for assurance that ultimately everything will be OK. So is the rest of the family.
- Graciously accept assistance from family, friends, and colleagues who offer to help. You will need it.
- Don't be afraid or ashamed to ask for psychological help for your loved one and for yourself. This is especially true when you become overwhelmed and feel helpless of your inability to comfort your loved one who often feels frustrated for many reasons.
- Make time to be present 24/7 at you loved one's bedside or for extended periods of the day. Your constant presence is a security blanket for your loved one. Make the evenings quality time for good conversation, listening to favorite music, reading to your loved one, or simply watch TV shows or movies.
- Engage in therapy sessions. Celebrate the "hallelujah moments" no matter how small the progress might be. Be the world's greatest cheerleader!! Applaud! Praise! Give high fives! Give a kiss and a hug. Any or all are great reinforcements for achievement and improvement.
- Keep a journal and make entries of the events of the day. It preserves time. Encourage everyone who visits to comment on everyday things like weather, current events, celebrity gossip, and other areas of interest in their journal entries. It helps patients feel as though they haven't lost time during recovery. These journal entries can be a mixed bag—very candid, reassuring, entertaining, and sometimes emotional.

- Decorate the hospital room with cards, stuffed animals, photographs, and flowers. Selina's friends made framed collages of photographs of friends and family and her pet dog in happier times. They were strategically placed where she could see them and reflect on happier times. Selina's little cousins also made and displayed special cards in the room, posted valentine window stickers, decorated eggs, and made Easter baskets.
- Attend the support group sessions conducted by hospital staff designed for family members and patients. They provide an understanding of normal brain function vs. the effects caused by injury/trauma, what recovering patients experience and what kind of emotional support they need.
- Take your loved ones outside to a garden when the weather is good. Get involved in recreational activities.
- If the patient has a pet, find ways to give them time to interact.
- Celebrate special days while in hospital (birthdays, holidays, etc.). These occasions recreate happier family moments and make hospital stays less gloomy.
- Make it a family event when the patient receives a day pass to go home for a Sunday visit. This is extremely meaningful to the patient's self worth and frame of mind. It is always a joy to go home!

The Learning Curve of Life After Brain Injury
Theresa M. Rankin

The coastal California newspaper, *The Cambrian* (Hearst Corporation), reported a front page story on May 12, 1977: "2 Badly Hurt When Car Goes over Hwy 1 Cliff. Two persons remained in serious condition Wednesday, five days after their new Porsche sports car plunged off a cliff . . . at a sharp curve along Pacific Coast Hwy 1."

The caption on the 1977 news photo of the wrecked sports car says, "A couple from San Diego was critically injured . . . when their new car plummeted from Hwy 1...The vehicle sailed across a 75-foot-space before plowing into a jutting headland and dropping to the beach."

I lost my life that day, May 5, 1977, as the passenger in a Porsche that careened off the cliffs of Pacific Coast Hwy 1. The story is mine only because I have a photograph of the crashed car resting on a rocky beach located north of Hearst Castle, San Simeon, California. When you look closely at the photograph, you will see that we are still in the car. "In the five seconds it took a gleaming new Porsche to plunge off the bluffs north of San Simeon, Theresa Rankin's carefully orchestrated life was rearranged like a suit of cards instantly shuffled," the story said.

Meg McConahey was the *Cambrian* reporter who wrote my story in 1982 when I returned to the scene to learn about the high-speed car crash that forever altered my life. The California Highway Patrol reported in its investigation that the driver of the Porsche, a naval flight officer based in San Diego, "approached a sharp-right hand curve at excessive speed. The Porsche, with only 558 miles on its odometer, crossed the southbound lane, the driver overcorrected, with his car crossing both lanes and up an inside embankment on the upland side of the road. The sports car then came off the embankment and again crossed the roadway at a second right hand curve. At that point the expensive, high-powered vehicle sailed off the cliff, traveled 75 feet across a cove and slammed broadside into a jutting cliff. The car dropped to the beach, rolled over several times and came to a stop on its wheels facing in the opposite direction, only a few feet from a receding high tide."

There were several miracles in those first few hours and days: Alex McLachlan, a resident of San Luis Obispo, was the first on the crash scene. Alex would serve not only as a first responder, but also as a photographer while he stood watch for the Cambria ambulance en route to the site. The next person to arrive on the isolated stretch of coastal highway was a nurse who knew a paramedic team was onsite at the Cambria Fire Department. "A protective ring of lifesavers began to collect, including the Cambria Ambulance crew and Scoop Morgan of the *Cambrian,* who captured the event on film," the article continued.

My story of triumph over tragedy involves nearly 30 years of fighting for access to healthcare critically needed to rebuild my life. The "learning curve" is truly about learning how to champion our right to access services and supports designed as person-centered and community-based.

I am a survivor of a traumatic brain injury (TBI). I carry both the duty and the responsibility to change the systemic barriers that stand in our way to equal access and appropriate healthcare services. We are a community of knowledge experts and advocates whose lives are as meaningful as the famous who survive such catastrophic injuries like Bob Woodruff and Christopher Reeve.

The tragedy was not as much about the car crash as it was about the total lack of comprehensive services and supports for the Theresa Rankin who survived a severe brain injury. My life was held in limbo for nearly nine years because there was no one to guide my Marine Corps family during the early stage of acute and post-acute medical care. My "life after brain injury" really began in April 1986. Then it became the journey of recovery. Amazing. That is the best word to describe the truth of how my referral to National Rehabilitation Hospital (NRH) actually came about. My father was reading a magazine in a dentist's office in Wisconsin, and there was an article about a craniofacial injury specialist in Bethesda, Maryland.

That dentist advised my father to find a way to bring me to Washington, D.C. for an evaluation by the craniofacial specialist mentioned in the article. That's what my father did. The specialist then referred me to NRH. I was suffering from severe and chronic muscleoskeletal injuries and chronic pain. He thought I needed a solid orthopedic evaluation and assessment by a physiatrist and physical therapist.

Amazing. I am the daughter of two U.S. Marines, and I know first-hand the long journey of recovery and community reintegration after trauma. My father, Chief Warrant Officer-4 Virgil Rankin, was my lifeline during this long period of rehabilitation because he knew the challenges of life after brain injury. He had survived two brain injuries. First, as child, he suffered a skull fracture and concussion when he was hit by a car while roller-skating in Washington, D.C. A second head injury occurred during his days as a U.S. Marine during the Korean War.

I believe we learn our survival skills as a young child. I believe we learn the skills of social navigation as a young adult. I believe my life prepared me to survive and thrive after experiencing a severe brain injury and the accompanying devastating cognitive impairments.

Today, I am a cofounder of Brain Injury Services, Inc., a national model of community-based services, advocacy, and supports for individuals and families coping with disability due to acquired and traumatic brain injuries. Today, I am also the National Community Educator and originator of BrainLine.org, a national public broadcasting multimedia project designed to provide trusted information on preventing, treating, and living life after brain injury. WETA Public TV 26 and the Defense and Veterans Brain Injury Center are leading the way in expanding the BrainLine project from its current

Website to a national outreach and education initiative. BrainLine is telling the powerful human stories of recovery, resilience, and reintegration after experiencing trauma, especially traumatic brain injury and post-traumatic stress disorder (PTSD.)

My Marine Corps family had no one to guide or counsel them during my long road to recovery. They searched for help and struggled to gain access for me to appropriate and comprehensive rehabilitation services. Today, military and civilian families are coping with levels of stress and hardship unlike any other time in our nation's history. This is our opportunity to harness the power of our stories, to take the lessons learned and to make a global difference as loved ones return home with forever altered lives.

I know all too well about the anger, frustration, grief, poverty, and helplessness brain-injured people can feel as they go on the difficult quest for a second chance at life. I also know the power in the kindness of strangers, and the power that results from developing a trusting relationship with your rehabilitation team. I found a lifesaving "circle of trust" at NRH when I arrived in Washington, D.C., after searching for advocacy and rehabilitation for almost nine years.

Still, many people who suffer brain injury struggle to find an answer to that critical question: Whom can we trust? Whom can we trust to understand the invisible pain we feel to understand the profound isolation we suffer and to understand the often invisible and debilitating disability caused by cognitive, visual, and auditory impairments? The journey of surviving a traumatic brain injury comes in many phases. With each phase of rehabilitation comes the chance to explore new and promising practices of recovery and resiliency.

Today, I chose not to write about my broken bones or to make a list of the impairments that affect my daily life. That's because the truth is my story is not about the burdens caused by brain injury, but about my mastery of a new life, my value as a knowledge expert, and my ongoing dreams and goals as a national community educator.

I hope you will join me on the journey to share knowledge and share lessons learned. I welcome your thoughts and ideas. I'm interested in learning who you are and what your journey is about at info@brainline.org. At BrainLine.org we are building a global story of triumph over tragedy, and I hope you will visit www.brainline.org and take advantage of what it offers.

Ferocious Advocates: The Griswold's Work to Change Their Son's World

Maryann Griswold

Chris Griswold and his best buddy, Joe, were driving home from a night out and a game of pool. The guys had grown up together in a close knit neighborhood in Waldorf, Maryland, more like brothers than friends. That night the streets were wet from an April rain and just blocks from home, the car spun out, skidded across the double yellow lines and struck a parked car. Chris and Joe, each just 24-years-old, were in critical condition. Joe wasn't expected to recover.

"I had fallen asleep on the sofa with a bad headache after work. Then at 2 a.m., a police officer came to our door," remembers Chris's mom, Maryann. "He told me there had been a terrible accident and that Chris had been taken to the ER at Civista Medical Center, and that he wasn't breathing on his own. He was being transported to the Washington Hospital Center, the officer said. All along, I thought he was in his room asleep."

The Griswold family's drive to the hospital on the morning of April 27, 2008, would be the beginning of a months' long odyssey through the healthcare system in search of the best care for Chris. His parents—always his loving supporters—became his strident advocates, fighting his battles when he could not.

When the family was finally allowed to see Chris, they reported, "He was in a coma. He had all kinds of tubes in his body, and a trachea tube was helping him breathe," Maryann says. "The doctors said it didn't look good. But I knew my son and I told them that he would pull through."

The Griswolds surrounded Chris with family and friends who gathered immediately to provide support. Maryann took a leave of absence from work and spent hours each day with Chris. Every day while he was in a coma, family and friends exercised his legs and arms. Maryann learned how to suction his trachea tube. "We didn't want to leave him alone for a minute. So many people love him and I wanted him to feel that," Maryann says. Then on May 8, Maryann's birthday wish for herself came true when Chris opened his eyes. "It was just for a moment, but we were all there, and it was the best gift I could have ever gotten."

By early June, the Griswolds were told to search for a place to send Chris—a nursing facility with rehabilitation services. They found a facil-

ity close to home and Chris was transferred. With no available room on
the rehab unit, Chris was put on the second floor, an inappropriate
placement that would prove disastrous.

"It was a nightmare," says Maryann. "He couldn't talk or move. There
was very little help, and he wasn't receiving any therapy. I was so afraid
to leave him alone, but I had to go back to work, so my good friend Dee,
who is like a second mom to Chris, went in my place. She was afraid at
first, but after she saw Chris, she went every day in the hours when my
husband and I couldn't be there. What we all saw happening was so
upsetting. He wasn't getting the care he needed. I'd call it abuse. That's
when we began to document each incident: oxygen that wasn't working
properly, a feeding tube hanging free, his air mattress that collapsed, his
dirty room. And he was being medicated when he didn't need to be and
the drug was keeping him from waking up."

The Griswolds photographed errors and doggedly registered complaints with staff. They often went directly to the facility administrator
to get action taken on Chris' behalf. They spoke to state inspectors who
were investigating the nursing home.

"We were Christopher's brain, his voice, his hands and legs,"
Maryann says. After a month, the Griswolds had had enough. "I looked
at my husband and cried, 'You have to get him out of here.' "

His family knew he would never improve without intensive rehabilitation, and they were determined to get him into the right hospital.
While it was further away from home, they pushed to get him a room at
the National Rehabilitation Hospital (NRH). By then, the facility
administrator had ordered physicians to stop giving Chris the medication that was keeping him unresponsive. The Griswolds started getting
Chris up and out of bed and videotaped his progress to convince everyone that he was ready for rehabilitation. Finally in July, Chris left the
nursing home for NRH.

"We drove him ourselves, oxygen tank and all," says Maryann. "It was
paradise compared to where I had been," Chris says. Within three days,
he was already making remarkable progress. His trachea tube was
removed and he began an intense therapy program that kept him working for eight hours a day. "They made him dress every day. They made
him move. Made him learn how to take care of himself," Maryann says.
"Soon he was talking. And all the while, we still worked with Chris, too.
Lots of nights, we came with friends and family to take Chris out to dinner. He was making great progress. I began to call him my miracle boy."

Sadly, Chris's friend Joe had died soon after the accident. The doctors had warned the Griswolds to wait before telling Chris the news. But at NRH, his psychotherapist felt it was time to answer his persistent questions about the incident and tell him about Joe's death. It was a crushing blow. "I lost my best friend," Chris said. "I will never forget Joe. He will always be in my heart."

While grieving and devastated by the loss, Chris didn't give up. He fought to get back his life, and his family fought along with him. "If it hadn't been for my mom and dad taking care of me, I don't know what would have happened. They kept fighting for me and so I'll keep fighting for me," Chris says.

After a month at NRH, Chris came home. Another month of outpatient therapy followed. Today Chris is physically strong and fit. He is back at work repairing computers. Those complex details he can recall. It's his short-term memory that has been left impaired. But neither Chris nor his family is letting this difficulty stand in his way. He uses techniques he learned in therapy to help. "I write notes to help me remember details," he says. His dad showed him how to use public transportation to get to work with the help of simple notes that mark which bus and train he needs to take. But Chris is already planning for the day when he will drive again, and ultimately, like all young men, he is looking forward to moving into a place of his own.

Maryann knows that a brain injury as severe as Chris' affects his "body, mind, and spirit." But she and her family haven't modified their expectations for Chris' future. "He is still Chris—a loving young man who has always been in tune to people's feelings. He is my son, I love him, and there is nothing I wouldn't do for him." That devotion was truly tested after Chris' accident and proved practically invincible.

"I discovered that I could fight hard when I had to for my child, but that is how I was raised. You do anything to help family." One of 15 siblings, Maryann grew up in a family in which taking care of one another was second nature. "You've got to be there for your child—every second. And you need the support of friends and family. Their help is so critical. I tell people no matter what kind of tragedy someone you care about experiences you should reach out to help. Do something, anything to support them—food shopping or house cleaning. Show your love and appreciation. It means so much during hard times," she says. "I know I can't change the world," Maryann adds. "But I felt certain I could and would do all could to change my son's world."

Appendix A
Rating Scales

Agitated Behavior Scale

This scale is used to determine if a person with a traumatic brain injury is agitated and to quantify the degree of agitation for the purpose of monitoring interventions made during rehabilitation. There are 14 items evaluated and each is scored from 1 point to 4 points. One point is for normal and 4 is for severe. The 14 items assessed are:

- Short attention span, easy distractibility, inability to concentrate.
- Impulsive, impatient, low tolerance for pain or frustration.
- Uncooperative, resistant to care, demanding.
- Violent and/or threatening violence toward people or property.
- Explosive and/or unpredictable anger.
- Rocking, rubbing, moaning, or other self-stimulating behavior.
- Pulling at tubes, restraints, etc.
- Wandering from treatment areas.
- Restlessness, pacing, excessive movement.
- Repetitive behaviors, motor and/or verbal.
- Rapid, loud, or excessive talking.
- Sudden changes of mood.
- Easily initiated or excessive crying and/or laughter.
- Self-abusiveness, physical and/or verbal.

Glasgow Coma Scale

The Glasgow Coma Scale (GCS) is an objective scale used to assess patients after trauma. It provides a grading for level of neurological impairment. The initial GCS (at the scene of injury) is used as a predictor for recovery. The scores range from 3 points to 15 points. Thirteen points to fifteen points is considered mild traumatic brain injury (TBI); 9 points to 12 points is moderate; and 8 points or less is severe (coma).

Eye-Opening Response
- Spontaneous opening with blinking: 4 points
- To verbal stimuli, command, speech: 3 points
- To pain only (not applied to face): 2 points
- No response: 1 point

Verbal Response
- Oriented: 5 points
- Confused conversation, but able to answer questions: 4 points
- Inappropriate words: 3 points
- Incomprehensible speech: 2 points
- No response: 1 point

Motor Response
- Obeys commands for movement: 6 points
- Purposeful movement to painful stimulus: 5 points
- Withdraws in response to pain: 4 points
- Flexion in response to pain (decorticate posturing): 3 points
- Extension response in response to pain (decerebrate posturing): 2 points
- No response: 1 point

Appendix B
Brain Injury Resources

American Heart Association
(800) 242-8721
www.americanheart.org

American Stroke Association
(888) 4-STROKE
www.strokeassociation.org

Brain Injury Association of America
105 North Alfred Street
Alexandria, VA 22314
Phone: (703) 236-6000
Family Helpline: Toll Free: (800) 444-6443
www.biausa.org

BrainLine.org
WETA
2775 South Quincy Street
Arlington, VA 22206
(703) 998-2020
www.brainline.org

Defense and Veterans Brain Injury Center (DVBIC)
Building 1, Room B209
Walter Reed Army Medical Center
6900 Georgia Avenue NW
Washington, DC 20307-5001
(800) 870-9244
(202) 782-6345
www.dvbic.org

Head Injury Hotline
(206) 621-8558
www.headinjury.com

National Rehabilitation Hospital
102 Irving Street, NW
Washington, DC 20010
(202) 877-1000
www.nrhrehab.org/TBI

National Stroke Association
(800) STROKES
www.stroke.org

Appendix C
Resources for People
with Brain Tumors

National Cancer Institute
At the National Cancer Institute (NCI), (800-4-CANCER), information specialists are available to answer questions about primary and secondary brain tumors and send relevant NCI materials. Their website is also an excellent resource for information: http://cancer.gov/publications. The following are examples of some of the booklets they have available:
- Radiation Therapy and You: A Guide to Self-Help During Treatment
- Chemotherapy and You: A Guide to Self-Help During Treatment
- Helping Yourself During Chemotherapy: 4 Steps for Patients
- Eating Hints for Cancer Patients
- Understanding Cancer Pain
- Pain Control: A Guide for People with Cancer and Their Families
- Get Relief From Cancer Pain—Taking Part in Clinical Trials: What Cancer Patients Need to Know
- La quimioterapia y usted: Una guia de autoayuda durante el tratamieto del cancer (Chemotherapy and You: A Guide to Self-HelpDuring Treatment for Cancer)
- La radioterapi y usted: Una guia de autoayuda durante el tratamiento del cancer (Radiation Therapy and You: A Guide to Self-Help During Treatment)
- ¿En que consisten los esudios clinicos? Un folleto para los pacientes de cancer (What Are Clinical Trials All About? A Guide for Cancer Patients Living with Cancer)
- Taking Time: Support for People With Cancer and the People Who Care About Them
- Facing Forward Series:
  - Life After Cancer Treatment
  - Ways You Can Make a Difference in Cancer
- Advanced Cancer: Living Each Day
- When Cancer Recurs: Meeting the Challenge

American Brain Tumor Association
(847) 827-9910
(800) 886-2282
www.abta.org

National Brain Tumor Society
East Coast Office
   124 Watertown Street, Suite 2D
   Watertown, MA 02472
   (617) 924-9997
West Coast Office
   22 Battery Street, Suite 612
   San Francisco, CA 94111-5520
   (415) 834-9970
Patient Services: (800) 934-2873
Toll-free: (800) 770-8287
Angel Adventure: (866) 455-3214
www.tbts.org

National Brain Tumor Foundation
www.braintumor.org
(800) 770-8287

COPE Program (Connection of Personal Experiences)
Volunteers offer support through a sharing of mutual experiences via
telephone and email conversations. Opportunity to feel understood, val-
idate feelings, offer emotional release, gain perspective through another person's experience. Contact Director of Support Services at (800)
770-8287, ext 25 or vai email at support@tbts.org.

Share the Care
An organization that provides a model for group care giving so that the
burden does not fall on the shoulders of a single or a couple of individuals. It was inspired by the experience of the founder who was called on
to gather a group of friends to find a way to help another friend cope
with cancer. Their website is www.sharethecare.org.

Family Caregiver Alliance

A nonprofit organization that offers a wealth of information for families and friends caring for adults with chronic, disabling illnesses. Newsletters, fact sheets (many in Spanish and Chinese), online support groups, audio workshops, resource lists, policy updates, caregiver advice and more are available free of charge on their website, www.caregiver.org.

Glossary

Many terms that you hear on the Brain Injury Rehabilitation Unit may be unfamiliar to you. Here are a few to get you started, but if you hear anyone discussing something that you don't understand, please feel free to ask. We understand that some of our common medical/rehabilitation language may not be so commonplace to you.

Words and phrases in *italics* are defined elsewhere within this glossary.

Activities of daily living (ADLs): describes everyday activities of self management including feeding, grooming, bathing, dressing and toileting; these may also be referred to as daily living skills (DLS)

Agraphia: inability to write; related to problem in the brain

Alexia: inability to read; related to problem in the brain

Ambulation: walking; however, the term "wheelchair ambulation" may be used; this means getting around in a wheelchair (or wheelchair mobility)

Ankle Foot Orthotic (AFO): a brace that helps with positioning a foot and ankle during standing, transfers, and walking

Anomia: the impaired ability to name objects or retrieve words

Agnosagnosia: an inability to realize (unawareness) one has a medical disorder or deficits in functioning

Anoxia: a lack of oxygen that can cause damage to brain cells; this condition can occur when blood flow to the brain is decreased

Aphasia: having problems understanding what people are saying or not being able to speak words; acquired as a result of a brain injury or stroke

Apraxia: not being able to make movements needed to do such things as speaking, moving arms and legs, walking, and dressing despite adequate strength to perform the tasks

Arousal: general state of alertness

Aspiration: the action of food or fluid entering the airway where it may remain or gradually move into the lungs; this may cause a person to choke or cough and may lead to an infection in the lungs (aspiration pneumonia)

Assistive Device/Assistive Equipment: equipment or devices, such as wheelchairs, braces, walkers or speech aids, that help a person perform activities of daily living

Attention: ability to concentrate; attention span is the length of time a person can concentrate on one task for a given period of time

Augmentative/Alternative Communication ("Aug Comm" or "AAC"): a system that helps people communicate with others (e.g., communication board, gestures, keyboard)

Benefits: services, procedures, or equipment for which a health insurance company will pay

Bivalve Cast: *a serial cast,* generally fiberglass or plaster that has been cut into two halves and is usually worn by the patient while in bed; these help maintain flexibility in the limb

Case Manager: a professional who works for a hospital, insurance company, or rehabilitation facility to make sure that all aspects of treatment comply with the rules of an individual's health insurance plan

Catheterization ("cath"): insertion of a small tube into the bladder to empty or collect urine; this tube may be left in the bladder (e.g., Foley catheter) or may be inserted intermittently; an alternative is external catheterization in which a collection device is applied to the penis (condom catheter)

Cognition (or cognitive): relating to mental functions of attention, memory, awareness, concentration, reasoning, judgment, understanding, etc.

Contracture: the inability of a joint to move due to soft tissue or bony limitations

Craniectomy: surgical removal of a portion of the skull to relieve pressure on the brain

Cranioplasty: surgically replacing the skull (or a plate) after *craniectomy*

Craniotomy: opening the skull to gain access to the brain (e.g., to remove blood, tumor, etc.) without removing the skull

CSF (Cerebrospinal fluid): a clear fluid that surrounds the brain and spinal cord and serves as a cushion to help protect the brain from injury

CT Scan (computed tomography scan; "CAT scan"): a noninvasive imaging technique that allows one to examine the brain and other organs through x-ray

Custodial Care: care that is provided to help patients take care of their daily needs (e.g., eating bathing, dressing, etc.) that does not require treatment or services from specially trained professionals, such as doctors, therapists, or rehabilitation nurses

CVA (cerebrovascular accident): *stroke*

Decubitus ulcer: *pressure sore*

Disability: the restriction or inability to perform a skill or activity that results from impairment, illness or injury

Doppler ultrasound: a noninvasive procedure to assess blood flow to look for the presence of blood clots in the arms or legs

Durable Medical Equipment (DME): equipment that has a medical purpose and can be used repeatedly, and is appropriate for use in the home, such as wheelchairs, walkers, etc.

DVT (deep venous thrombosis): blood clot in a vein

Dysarthria: loss or impairment in the ability to speak clearly due to loss of motor control in the muscles to produce speech

Dysgraphia: difficulty writing

Dysphagia: difficulty swallowing

Edema: swelling

EEG (electroencephalograph): a test that measures the electrical activity in the brain, often used to detect seizure activity

Environmental Adaptations: modifications to a person's environment that enhances independence, such as ramps or elevators

Epilepsy: recurrent seizures

Flaccidity: loss or absence of muscle tone resulting in a limb feeling "floppy;" may make it difficult for patients to support themselves in a sitting or standing position. Flaccidity in the arm can result in *subluxation* or dislocation of a shoulder joint if the arm is not supported

Functional Ability: a person's ability to perform activities of daily living (eating, bathing, dressing, communicating, etc.) without help from another person

Hemianopsia: loss of vision in one-half of the visual field in one or both eyes; if the same visual field is lost in both eyes, it is referred to as a *homonomous hemianopsia*

Hemiparesis: weakness on one side of the body

Hemiplegia: *paralysis* on one side of the body

Heterotopic Ossification (HO): formation of bone in abnormal areas, such as muscles

Homonomous hemianopsia: loss of one-half of the visual field that results from loss of the same visual field in both eyes

Hydrocephalus: an excessive amount of cerebrospinal fluid in the brain causing increased pressure on, and possible damage to, brain tissue

Incontinence: having bowel or bladder accidents (continence is the ability to control bowel and bladder function voluntarily)

Lability: a brief or rapidly changing display of emotion (e.g., laughing, crying, etc.) with little or no provocation

Modified Barium Swallow (MBS): x-ray test performed by a speech language pathologist in conjunction with a radiologist where various consistencies of food and liquids are coated with barium so they can be seen on x-ray; the different foods/drinks are consumed by the patient and recorded on videocassette. Swallowing is assessed to determine the appropriate diet level and to assist with techniques to improve swallowing

Motor Control: the ability to use muscles to move a limb or other body part in a smooth and coordinated manner to complete a desired function

MRI (magnetic resonance imaging): computerized noninvasive imaging technique for viewing the organs and structures in the body, using a very powerful magnet; therefore, patients with pacemakers, metal in their body or certain other implantable medical devices probably cannot have this test

MVA: motor vehicle accident

Neglect: a person does not identify, process, or attend to things on one side of the body or environment; for example, one may ignore an arm or one side of the meal tray, however, this is not a result of loss of vision

Neurogenic bladder: abnormal functioning of the bladder due to disease or injury of the central nervous system (brain or spinal cord) or the peripheral nervous system

Neurogenic bowel: abnormal functioning of the bowel due to disease or injury of the central nervous system (brain or spinal cord) or the peripheral nervous system

Neurologist: a doctor who specializes in diagnosis and treatment of diseases of, or injuries to, the nervous system, including brain and spinal cord

Neuropsychologist: a licensed psychologist who has undergone specialized training to provided assessment and treatment for persons who have disorders of the nervous system, including brain and spinal cord

Neurotransmitters: chemicals made in the nervous system that serve as messengers throughout the nervous system aiding or interfering with the functions of nerve cells

NPO (an abbreviation meaning "nothing by mouth"): if a sign is posted in a patient's room indicating one is "NPO," then one should not be given any food, water or medication by mouth

Nursing Home (skilled nursing facility or SNF, often pronounced "snif"): a facility where patients stay to receive rehabilitation services, long-term care, or skilled nursing care

Nystagmus: a rapid, jerky movement of the eyes that occurs as the result of injury to the *vestibular system*

Occupational Therapist (OT): a rehabilitation professional who teaches skills and adaptations that allows people with disabilities to be as independent as possible with activities of daily living

Orientation: awareness of self, place, time, and situation

Orthoses (or orthotics): devices designed to support a weakened joint or limb

Outpatient Rehabilitation: rehabilitation services provided to person who lives at home; it may be a comprehensive, daily program of multiple services, or only one or two services a few times a week

Paralysis: the inability to move a part of one's body, such as an arm or leg

Paraplegia: paralysis of both legs

PEG tube (percutaneous gastrostomy tube): feeding tube; "G-tube"

Perception: the active process of receiving information from one's immediate surroundings through the five senses and immediately translating that information to meaning based on past experiences

Perseveration: repeating one word or phrase (verbal perseveration) or a motor task (motor perseveration) and unable to switch back to or progress on to another topic/task

Physiatrist: a doctor who specializes in physical medicine and rehabilitation

Physical Therapist (PT): a rehabilitation professional who works to restore one's movement abilities through improving motor control and adaptive techniques; this discipline concentrates on the motor control of the patient for functional activities such as transfers and walking

PO: abbreviation for "by mouth"

Post Traumatic Amnesia (PTA): a period of days, weeks, or months after the brain injury when the patient suffers a loss of day-to-day memory; the patient is unable to store new information and, therefore, has a decreased ability to learn; memory of the PTA period is never stored and things that happened during that period cannot be recalled

Pragmatics: ability to use language skills for social communication purposes (e.g., taking turns, maintaining topic, shifting topics, etc.)

Pressure sore (bed sore or decubitus ulcer): a reddened area or open skin wound caused by unrelieved pressure on the skin over bony areas such as the hip bone or tail bone, or areas of external pressure, such as a poorly fitting brace

PRN: abbreviation for "as needed"

Problem Solving: ability to evaluate a situation and come to appropriate solutions

Prostheses: artificial limbs or body parts

Quadriplegia: see *tetraplegia*

Range of Motion (ROM): The amount of movement at a joint, as measured in number of degrees; ROM is generally determined by the degree of flexibility of the muscles around the joint, although limitations may also occur as a result of bony limitations. ROM can be divided into active range of motion (AROM), which is how much range of motion the patient has without assistance, and passive range of motion (PROM), which is how far someone else can move a person's limb through a range of motion. AROM can also be affected by nerve damage and weakness despite a normal PROM

Reasoning: ability to think beyond the concrete (here and now) level; ability to mentally manipulate information to solve problems

Recreational Therapist (RT): therapists who use a wide range of recreational activities in both the hospital and community to improve the physical, social and leisure needs of persons with disabilities

Resting Hand Splint: a device made of molded plastic and held on with Velcro straps which hold the hand in a neutral position; the splint can be used to protect a *flaccid* hand from injury or to keep a hand that has increased tone *(spasticity)* in an extended position

Serial Cast: a cast put on by an occupational or physical therapist that is designed to help stretch out muscles which have become tight following an injury; these casts are often changed every five to seven days or they may be *bivalve casts* which are put on and taken off more frequently.

Seizure: abnormal electrical discharges in the brain which can cause any brief neurologic symptoms. Most commonly, there will be some alteration or loss of consciousness, but this is not necessary. Symptoms may range from staring spells to movement (e.g., jerking) in part of one limb, an entire limb, one side of the body, or all extremities

Social Worker: a professional who assists patients, families, and their significant others with psychosocial and environmental barriers that predispose illness or interfere with obtaining maximum benefit from medical and rehabilitation care; also assists with continued care planning that optimizes the patient's independence

Spasticity: increased muscle tone in a limb resulting in the feeling of the limb being too stiff/tight. Spasticity is "velocity dependent" so if the patient's limb is put through a slow range of motion, the spasticity may not be noticed; however, if the range is done at a higher velocity, it may become quite noticeable; this may make it more difficulty for a patient to move a limb and can also cause pain and difficulty with positioning

Speech-Language Pathologist (SLP): a rehabilitation professional who works to restore swallowing, communication, and cognitive skills

Status Epilepticus: a single seizure or multiple seizures without complete return to baseline between seizures, lasting more than 30 minutes

Stroke (CVA): a sudden interruption of blood flow to an area of the brain, caused by a blockage (e.g., a blood clot) or by bleeding (e.g., a hemorrhage)

Subacute Rehabilitation: rehabilitation services that include daily nursing care, supervision by a rehabilitation doctor, and medical care as needed; rehabilitation therapies are usually less intensive and the person's stay is typically longer than in acute rehabilitation

Subluxation: an incomplete dislocation

Tetraplegia (quadriplegia): weakness in all four limbs

Tone: the tension of a muscle at rest. Normal muscle tone increases with activity; following a brain injury, a person can have abnormal tone that is lower or higher than usual. (See *flaccidity* and *spasticity.*)

Tracheostomy tube ("trach"): the procedure of making an airway in the neck directly into the trachea (windpipe) and inserting a tube ("trach") through which the patient can breathe

Vertigo: dizziness; the feeling that one is spinning or that one's surroundings are spinning

Vestibular System: the part of the nervous system that is involved with balance; there is a peripheral portion that involves the middle and inner ear and the nerve tracking to the brainstem and also the central portion that involves the posterior portion of the brain (cerebellum or brainstem)

Visual Field Cut: the loss of vision in one portion of the person's visual field; often it is one half of the visual field (*hemianopsia*) or a quarter of a visual field (*quadrantanopsia*). Visual field cuts which result from injury to the brain lead to field cuts which are the same (or similar) in both eyes, in other words, a "right *homonomous hemianopsia*" involves the right field in both eyes; not just the right eye

Vocational Rehabilitation: services that help to determine a person's strengths and weaknesses and provide guidance for employment or educational planning

VP Shunt (ventriculoperitoneal shunt): a tube that drains excess *CSF* from the ventricles in the brain into the abdomen; used in the treatment of *hydrocephalus*

Weight-bearing: amount of weight a person can put through their extremities, usually after a fracture or surgical procedure to a limb; different grades of weight-bearing include:

NWB	Non weight-bearing
FFWB	Foot flat weight-bearing
PWB	Partial weight-bearing; the doctor will usually give a specific percentage of the weight that may be loaded on the limb.
TTWB	Toe-touch weight-bearing
WBAT	Weight-bearing as tolerated
FWB	Full weight-bearing

Reference Notes

Chapter 1

Bradley, W., Daroff, R., Fenichel, G., & Jankovic, J. (2008). *Neurology in Clinical Practice* (5th ed.). Philadelphia: Butterworth Heinemann Elsevier.

Duus, P. (1989). *Topical Diagnosis in Neurology* (2nd ed.). New York, NY: Thieme.

Netter, F. (1990). *Atlas of Human Anatomy.* Summit, NJ: Ciba-Geigy Corporation.

Nolte, J. (1993). *The Human Brain: An Introduction to Its Functional Anatomy.* St. Louis, MO: Mosby.

Zasler, N., Katz, D., & Zafonte, R. (2007). *Brain Injury Medicine: Principles and Practice.* New York: Demos.

Chapter 2

Bradley, W.G., Daroff, R.B., Fenichel, G.M., & Jankovic, J. (Eds.). (2008). *Neurology in Clinical Practice* (5th ed). Philadelphia, PA: Butterworth Heinemann-Elsevier.

Brazis, P., Masdeu, J., & Biller, J. (1996). *Localization in Clinical Neurology* (3rd ed.). Boston: Little, Brown & Company.

Gordon, W., Zafonte, R., Cicerone, K., & et al. (2006). Traumatic brain injury rehabilitation: State of the science. *American Journal of Physical Medicine & Rehabilitation*, 85, 343-382.

Greenberg, M. (2005). *Handbook of Neurosurgery.* New York, NY: Thieme Medical Publishers.

Rao, P.R., Conroy, B.E. & Baron, C. (Eds.). (2009). *Managing Stroke: A Guide to Living Well after Stroke* (2nd Ed.). Washington, DC: NRII Press.

Silver, J., McAllister, T., & Yudofsky, S. (2004). *Textbook of Traumatic Brain Injury.* Washington, DC: American Psychiatric Publishing, Inc.

Writing Group Members. (2009). Heart disease and stroke Statistics-2009 Update: A report from the American Heart Association statis tics Committee. *Circulation*. 119, c21-e181.

Zasler, N, Katz, D, & Zafonte, R (2007). *Brain Injury Medicine: Principles and Practice*. New York: Demos.

Chapter 3

National Institutes of Health, National Cancer Institute, US Dept of Health and Human Services, Public Health Service. (2002). *What You Need to Know about Brain Tumors* [NIH Publication No. 02-1558]. Bethesda, MD: Authors.

Information about brain tumors. Retrieved December 12, 2008, from National Brain Tumor Society Web site: http://www.tbts.org/TumorsSublanding.

What is palliative care? Retrieved January 31, 2009, from GetPalliativeCare.org Web site: http://www.getpalliativecare.org/whatis.

Armstrong, T., Cohen, M., Hess, K.R., & et al. (2006). Complementary and alternative medicine use and quality of life in patients with primary brain tumors. *Journal of Pain and Symptom Management*, 32, 148-154.

Davies, E., Hall, S., & Clarke, C. (2003). Two year survival after malignant cerebral glioma: Patient and relative reports of handicap, psychiatric symptoms and rehabilitation. *Journal of Pain and Symptom Management*, 25, 259-266.

Guo, Y., Young, B., Hainley, S., et al. (2007). Evaluation and pharmacologic management of symptoms in cancer patients undergoing acute rehabilitation in a comprehensive cancer center. *Archives of Physical Medicine and Rehabilitation*, 88, 891-895.

Janda, M., Steginga, S., Langbecker, D., et al. (2007). Quality of life among patients with a brain tumor and their careers. *Journal of Psychosomatic Research*, 63, 617-623.

Keir, S., Swartz, J., & Friedman, H. (2007). Stress and long-term survivors of brain cancer. *Support Care Cancer*, 15, 1423-1428.

Schmer, C., Ward-Smith, P., Latham, S., & Salacz, M. (2008). When a family member has a malignant brain tumor: The caregiver perspective. *Journal of Neuroscience Nursing*, 40, 1975-1984.

Sherwood, P.R., Given, B.A., Given, C.W., & et al. (2006). .Predictors of distress in caregivers of persons with a primary malignant brain tumor. *Research in Nursing & Health*, 29, 105-120.

Weitzner, M. A. Meyers, C. A. , & Byrne, K. (1996). Psychosocial functioning and quality of life in patients with primary brain tumors. *Journal of Neurosurgy*, 84, 29-34.

Chapter 4

High W., Sander A., Struchen M., & Hart K. (2005). *Rehabilitation for Traumatic Brain Injury.* New York: Oxford University Press.

Scheiman, M. (2002). *Understanding and Managing Vision Deficits: A Guide for Occupational Therapists.* (2nd ed.). Slack Incorporated

Senelick, R. & Cougherty, K. (2001). *Living with Brain Injury: A Guide for Families.* (2nd edition). Birmingham, AL: HealthSouth Press.

Umphred, D. (2001). *Neurological Rehabilitation.* (4th ed). St. Louis: Mosby.

Zoltan, Barbara. (1996). *Vision, Perception, and Cognition: A Manual for the Evaluation and Treatment of the Neurologically Impaired Adult.* (3rd ed.). Thorofare, NJ: Slack Incorporated.

Chapter 5

American Speech-Language-Hearing Association. (2001). *Let's Talk: Cognitive-Communication Problems Following Right Hemisphere Damage.* Rockville, MD: Cherney, L.

American Speech-Language-Hearing Association. (2001). *Let's Talk: Brain Injury.* Rockville, MD: Gillis, R.

American Speech-Language-Hearing Association. (2001). *Let's Talk: Dysarthria.* Rockville, MD: Yorkston, K.

Baylor College of Medicine. (2002). *Picking Up the Pieces after TBI: A Guide for Family Members.* Houston, TX: Sander, A.M.

National Institute on Deafness and Other Communication Disorders. (1998). *Fact Sheet - Traumatic Brain Injury: Cognitive and Communication Disorders.* Bethesda, MD.

National Institute on Deafness and Other Communication Disorders. (1998). *Fact Sheet - Dysphagia.* Bethesda, MD.

Sohlberg, M.M. & Mateer, C. (1989). *Introduction to Cognitive Rehabitation: Theory & Practice.* New York, NY: The Guilford Press.

Chapter 6

Riley, G. A. (2007). Stress and depression in family carers following traumatic brain injury: the influence of beliefs about difficult behaviours. *Clinical Rehabilitation*, 21(1), 82-88.

Winkler, D., Unsworth, C., & Sloan, S. (2006). Factors that lead to successful community integration following severe traumatic brain injury. *Journal of Head Trauma Rehabilitation*, 21(1), 8-21.

Chapter 7

Keefe, S. (2007). Catch a falling star: Fall prevention program shines at JFK/Johnson Rehab Institute. *ADVANCE for Physical Therapists and PT Assistants*, 11-13.

Rao, P.R., Conroy, B.E. & Baron, C. (Eds.). (2009). *Managing Stroke: A Guide to Living Well after Stroke* (2nd Ed.). Washington, DC: NRH Press.

Tinnetti, M. (2003). Preventing falls in elderly persons. *New England Journal of Medicine*, 348(1): 42-49.

Chapter 8

(2001). Antiseizure prophylaxis for penetrating brain injury. *Journal of Trauma Injury, Infection and Critical Care*, 51, S41-S43.

Ballesteros, J., Itziar, G, Ibarra, N, & Quemada, J (2008). The effectiveness of donepezil for cognitive rehabilitation after traumatic brain injury: A systematic review. *Journal Head Trauma Rehabilitation*, 23(3), 171-180.

Chang, B., & Lowenstein, D. (2003). Practice parameter: Antiepileptic drug prophylaxis in severe traumatic brain injury: Report of the Quality Standards Subcommittee of the American Academy of Neurology. *Neurology*, 60, 10-16.

Elovic, E., Jasey, N., & Eisenberg, M. (2008). The use of atypical antipyschotics after traumatic brain injury. *Journal of Head Trauma Rehabilitation*, 23(2), 132-135.

Elovic, E. (2000).Use of Provigil for underarousal following TBI. *Journal of Head Trauma Rehabilitation*, 15(4), 1068-1071.

Gordon, W., Zafonte, R., Cicerone, K., & et al. (2006). Traumatic brain injury rehabilitation. *American Journal of Physical Medicine and*

Rehabilitation, 85, 343-382.

Lew, H., Fuh, J., Wang, S., & et al. (2006). Characteristics and treatment of headache after traumatic brain injury. *American Journal of Physical Medicine and Rehabilitation*, 619-627.

Lu, B., & Zee, P. (2006). Circadian rhythm sleep disorders. *Chest*, 130, 1915-1923.

O'Shankick, G. (2006). Update on antidepressants. *Journal of Head Trauma Rehabilitation*, 21(3), 282-284.

Retrieved March 12, 2009, from Epocrates.com Web site: http://www.epocrates.com.

Retrieved March 27, 2009, from Physicians Drug Reference Online Web site: http://www.pdr.net.

Silver, J., Koumaras, B., Chen, M., & et al. (2006). Effects of rivastigmine on cognitive function in patients with traumatic brain injury. *Neurology*, 67, 748-755.

Waldon-Perrine, R., Hanks, R., & Perrine, S. (2008). Pharmacotherapy for postacute traumatic brain injury: A literature review for guidance in psychological practice. *Rehabilitation Psychology*, 53(4), 426-444.

Chapter 9

Media Partners, Inc. (2005). Introduction to *Acquired Brain Injury: A Family Guide to Understanding Traumatic Brain Injury, Stroke, Aneurysm, and the Early Recovery Process*. Media Partners, Inc.: Duluth, Georgia.

Sander, A. (2002). *Picking Up the Pieces after TBI: A Guide for Family Members*. Baylor College of Medicine: Houston, Texas.

Struchen, M.A., West, D., Cannon, N., Eckenrode, L., Backrus, P, Jaffrey, S., Gautreau, M., Caroselli, J., & Keenan, L. (2006). *Making Connections after Brain Injury: A Guide for Social Peer Mentors*. Baylor College of Medicine: Houston, Texas.

Taylor, Ll, & Kreutzer, J. (2003). How to talk to children about brain injury. *TBI Today*, Vol. 1, #3. Virginia Commonwealth University: Richmond, Virginia.

The National Resource Center for Traumatic Brain Injury (1999). *Getting Better and Better after Brain Injury: A Guide for Families, Friends, and Caregivers for Living Smarter and Happier*. Virginia Commonwealth University: Richmond, Virginia.

Chapter 10

Corrigan, J. D., Smith-Knapp, K., & Granger, C. V. (1998). Outcomes in the first 5 years after traumatic brain injury. *Archives of Physical Medicine and Rehabilitation,* 79, 298-305.

DSM-IV-TR: Diagnostic and Statistical Manual of Mental Disorders, Text Revision (4th edition) (2000). Washington, DC: American Psychiatric Association.

Heinemann, A. W., Corrigan, J. D., & Moore, D. (2004). Case management for traumatic brain injury survivors with alcohol problems. *Rehabilitation Psychology,* 49 (2), 156-166.

Jorge, R. E., Robinson, R. G., et al. (2004). Major depression following traumatic brain injury. *Archives of General Psychiatry,* 61, 42-50.

Maier, R. V. (2005). Controlling alcohol problems among hospitalized trauma patients. *The Journal of Trauma,* 59, S1-S2.

Miller, N. A., & Adams, J. (2005). Alcohol and drug disorders. In Silver, J. M., McAllister, T. W., & Yudofsky, S. C., *Textbook of Traumatic Brain Injury.* Washington, DC: American Psychiatric Publishing, Inc.

Newman, A. C., Garmoe, W., Beatty, P., & Ziccardi, M. (2000). Self-awareness of traumatically brain injured patients in the acute inpatient rehabilitation setting. *Brain Injury,* 14(4), 333-344.

Chapter 11

sexuality. (n.d.). *The American Heritage® Dictionary of the English Language,* Fourth Edition. Retrieved December 04, 2008, from Dictionary.com website:
http://dictionary.reference.com/browse/sexuality

Griffith, E. R. & Lemberg, S. (1993). *Sexuality and the Person with Traumatic Brain Injury: A Guide for Families.* Philadelphia: F. A. Davis

Rolland, J. S. (1994). *Families, Illness, and Disability: An Integrative Treatment Model.* New York: Harper Collins Publishers, Inc.

Chapter 12

Bunch, J. (2000). *Young Adults with Brain Injury and College. TBI Challenge,* 4 (2), 5.

Office for Civil Rights. (2005, March 10). Retrieved September 7, 2007,

from U.S Department of Education:
http://ed.gov/about/offices/list/ocr/docs/auxaids.html.

Da Silva-Cardosa, E., Romero, M., Chan, F., & et al. (2007). Disparities in vocational rehabilitation services and outcomes for Hispanic clients with traumatic brain injury: Do they exist? *Journal of Head Trauma Rehabilitation*, 22 (2), 85-94.

Fadyl, J., & McPherson, K. (2009). Approaches to vocational rehabilitation after traumatic brain injury: A review of the evidence. *Journal of Head Trauma Rehabilitation*, 24 (3), 195-212.

The Student with a Brain Injury: Achieving Goals for Higher Education. (n.d.). Retrieved October 2007, from Heath Resource Center: www.heath-resource-center.org.

Todis, B., & Glang, A. (2008). Redefining success: Results of a qualitative study of postsecondary transition outcomes for youth with traumatic brain injury. *Journal Head Trauma Rehabilitation*, 23 (4), 252-263.

U.S. Department of Education. (2007, March). Retrieved September 7, 2007, from Office for Civil Rights: http://www.ed.gov/about/offices/list/ocr/transition.html.

U.S. Department of Justice Americans with Disability Act (2009, July). Retrieved July 16, 2009, from ADA Home Page: http://www.ada.gov.

Wehman, P., Targett, P., Yasuda, S., & et al. (2007). Helping persons with traumatic brain injury of minority origin: Improve career and employment outcomes. *Journal of Head Trauma Rehabilitation*, 22 (2), 95-104.

Chapter 13

Burlingame, J. & Skalko, T. K. (1997). *Idyll Arbor's Glossary for Therapists.* Enumclaw, WA: Idyll Arbor.

Carter, M. J., Van Andel, G. E. & Robb, G. M. (1995). *Therapeutic Recreation a Practical Approach* (2nd ed.). Long Grove, IL: Waveland Press.

Falvo, Donna R. (1999). *Medical and Psychosocial Aspects of Chronic Illness and Disability* (2nd ed.). Gaithersburg, MD: Aspen Publication.

Retrieved March 26, 2009, from Therapeutic Recreation Directory Online Web site: http://www.recreationtherapy.com.

Index